D1201455

Karen A. Theesen, PharmD

The Handbook
of Psychiatric Drug Therapy
for Children and Adolescents

Pre-publication
REVIEWS,
COMMENTARIES,
EVALUATIONS . . .

"**D**r. Theesen's *The Handbook of Psychiatric Drug Therapy for Children and Adolescents* is the best compilation of literature and clinical wisdom of using psychotherapeutic drugs in children and adolescents. For each category of drugs, specific information is included regarding efficacy, developmental pharmacokinetic differences and dosing recommendations in younger and older children, adverse effects reported in children, as well as detailed yet practical monitoring guidelines which include needed baseline assessments and specific instructions for parents or caregivers. Each section provides comprehensive references. This volume is a valuable reference for all clinicians who treat or counsel children and adolescents given psychotherapeutic drugs."

Glen L. Stimmel, PharmD
Professor of Clinical Pharmacy and Psychiatry,
University of California Schools of Pharmacy and Medicine

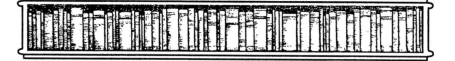

"**P**sychopharmacology for children and adolescents emerges from two young disciplines–child psychiatry and psychopharmacology. Dr. Theesen combines contemporary literature and research from both fields in an easy to read and use text. This book is a must for both child fellows and practitioners who wish to use and understand contemporary treatments. Dr. Theesen reviews the 'tried and true' medications useful for children and adolescents as well as the findings emerging from new research on psychopharmacology in youth."

Elissa P. Benedek, MD
Director, Research and Training Center for Forensic Psychiatry; Clinical Professor of Psychiatry, University of Michigan

"**T**his resource is worth the price for the section bibliographies alone. The author reviews the published study and case literature on the use of psychotropic agents in children and adolescents. Unfortunately, there are more questions than answers when it comes to use of these agents in the pediatric population, and the author frequently acknowledges this fact. This book will be a useful pocket resource to give brief product information including approval status in children (by the FDA and United States Pharmacopeia), trade names and generic availability, and the average wholesale price. It also gives information on dosage ranges that have been used in children, recommendations for baseline and follow-up monitoring parameters, a review of adverse drug effect reports involving children, and an overview of instructions for patients and their caregivers.

We all must acknowledge the lack of well-controlled studies to evaluate the use of psychotropic agents in this population; again, children must be recognized as the 'therapeutic orphans' that they are. However, this handbook will give clinicians useful information to consider as they treat children and adolescents with depression, anxiety, attention deficit disorder, enuresis, obsessive-compulsive disorder, bipolar disorder, and psychosis."

Linda K. Ohri, PharmD
Manager, Pediatric Drug Information Service, Children's Hospital, Omaha, NE; Assistant Professor, Creighton University School of Pharmacy and Allied Health Professions

More pre-publication
REVIEWS, COMMENTARIES, EVALUATIONS . . .

"This book is exceptionally thorough in its coverage of psychopharmacological agents that are utilized for children and adolescents. The summary review of research in each chapter that covers a specific category of medication is very helpful for the clinician in targeting symptoms and evaluating specific behavioral outcomes of pharmacological treatment. The research reviews also clearly illustrate the need for further research in the area of psychopharmacological treatment of children and adolescents.

Extensive information about common side effects and those peculiar to children and adolescents will be particularly helpful to nurses in assessing the child's response to medication therapy. In addition, information on interactions with other classes of drugs is useful as the drugs may affect normal growth and development.

This book is a valuable resource for clinicians of all educational backgrounds who work with children and adolescents in psychiatric/mental health, educational, or rehabilitation settings."

Stephanie Stockard Spelic, RN
Assistant Professor of Psychiatric Mental Health Nursing, Creighton University School of Nursing

"Dr. Theesen has written a comprehensive handbook on psychopharmacotherapy for children and adolescents that is organized, succinct, and up to date. It is addressed not only to physicians but also to other health care professionals who treat psychiatrically ill children.

With this handbook, I no longer need to review any other references to feel comfortable in prescribing and maintaining a child/adolescent on psychotherapeutic drugs. The most helpful sections for myself in a busy private practice setting have been monitoring guidelines, drug interactions, and contraindications. Regarding time constraints that mean it is not always possible to review recent literature, Dr. Theesen has done this already in sections on studies of efficacy and case reports. This handbook is a must for anyone treating psychiatrically ill children."

Marilou Woodard, MD
Child and Adolescent Psychiatrist; Medical Director of Therapeutic Foster Care, Methodist Richard Young Center, Omaha, NE

Pharmaceutical Products Press
An Imprint of the Haworth Press, Inc.

The Handbook
of Psychiatric Drug Therapy
for Children and Adolescents

PHARMACEUTICAL PRODUCTS PRESS
Pharmaceutical Sciences
Mickey C. Smith, PhD
Executive Editor

New, Recent, and Forthcoming Titles:

Principles of Pharmaceutical Marketing edited by Mickey C. Smith

Pharmacy Ethics edited by Mickey C. Smith, Steven Strauss, John Baldwin, and Kelly T. Alberts

Drug-Related Problems in Geriatric Nursing Home Patients by James W. Cooper

Pharmacy and the U.S. Health Care System edited by Jack E. Fincham and Albert I. Wertheimer

Pharmaceutical Marketing: Strategy and Cases by Mickey C. Smith

International Pharmaceutical Services: The Drug Industry and Pharmacy Practice in Twenty-Three Major Countries of the World edited by Richard N. Spivey, Albert I. Wertheimer, and T. Donald Rucker

A Social History of the Minor Tranquilizers: The Quest for Small Comfort in the Age of Anxiety by Mickey C. Smith

Marketing Pharmaceutical Services: Patron Loyalty, Satisfaction, and Preferences edited by Harry A. Smith and Joel Coons

Nicotine Replacement: A Critical Evaluation edited by Ovide F. Pomerleau and Cynthia S. Pomerleau

Herbs of Choice: The Therapeutic Use of Phytomedicinals by Varro E. Tyler

Interpersonal Communication in Pharmaceutical Care by Helen Meldrum

Searching for Magic Bullets: Orphan Drugs, Consumer Activism, and Pharmaceutical Development by Lisa Ruby Basara and Michael Montagne

The Honest Herbal by Varro E. Tyler

Understanding the Pill: A Consumer's Guide to Oral Contraceptives by Greg Juhn

Pharmaceutical Chartbook, Second Edition edited by Abraham G. Hartzema and C. Daniel Mullins

The Handbook of Psychiatric Drug Therapy for Children and Adolescents by Karen A. Theesen

Children, Medicines, and Culture edited by Patricia J. Bush, Deanna J. Trakas, Emilio J. Sanz, Alan Prout, Tuula Vaskilampi, and Rolf L. Wirsing

The Handbook
of Psychiatric Drug
Therapy
for Children
and Adolescents

Karen A. Theesen, PharmD

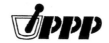

Pharmaceutical Products Press
An Imprint of the Haworth Press, Inc.
New York • London

Published by

Pharmaceutical Products Press, an imprint of The Haworth Press, Inc., 10 Alice Street, Binghamton, NY 13904-1580

Theesen, Karen A.
    The handbook of psychiatric drug therapy for children and adolescents / Karen A. Theesen.
        p.   cm.
    Includes bibliographical references and index.
    ISBN 1-56024-929-3 (alk. paper)
    1. Pediatric psychopharmacology–Handbooks, manuals, etc. I. Title.
    [DNLM: 1. Psychotropic Drugs–pharmacology. 2. Drug Therapy–in infancy & childhood. 3. Drug Therapy–in adolescence. 4. Psychotropic Drugs–therapeutic use. QV 77.2 T375h 1995]
RJ504.7.T44   1995
618.92'8918–dc20
DNLM/DLC
for Library of Congress   95-8194
                                                                                                 CIP

To my nieces and nephew:
Melissa, Brandee, and Ross Theesen

ABOUT THE AUTHOR

Karen A. Theesen, PharmD, is Associate Professor of Pharmacy and Psychiatry at Creighton University in Omaha, Nebraska. Dr. Theesen is a practitioner at the St. Joseph Center for Mental Health. She is the Formulary Consultant for the Department of Institutions for the State of Nebraska and is a member of the Expert Advisory Panel in Psychiatry for the USP. Dr. Theesen is a Past President of the Nebraska Society of Health-System Pharmacists.

CONTENTS

Preface

The purpose of *The Handbook of Psychiatric Drug Therapy for Children and Adolescents* is to provide the user with current information on the safety and efficacy of the psychotropic agents in the pediatric population. This handbook provides information on the pharmacokinetics, adverse effects, dosing, and suggested monitoring guidelines for children and adolescents, and serves as an excellent reference to the practitioner. *The Handbook of Psychiatric Drug Therapy for Children and Adolescents* avoids repeating or extrapolating the adult information on indications, adverse effects, dosing, etc. It is assumed that any adverse effect that has been reported in adults may occur in children and adolescents, sooner or later. What is unknown for many drugs is what adverse effects occur in the developing child or adolescent and are not found in the adult population. Only the drugs that have been used to treat disorders in children and adolescents are included in this text; therefore, not all psychotropic agents are included.

Much more research is needed in the entire area of child and adolescent psychopharmacology. Most of the studies of psychotropic drug therapy in children and adolescents involve less than 20 patients and are not double-blind or placebo controlled. For some drugs, the number of cases reported with adverse effects exceeds the number of patients reported with a positive effect. Practitioners are encouraged to prescribe limited amounts of these medications to all patients due to the significant risk of toxicity in overdose. Following each of the proposed DSM-IV (Diagnostic and Statistical Manual of Mental Disorders, Fourth Edition) indications for the use of the psychotropics is one or more question marks. The number of question marks reflects the lack of information in this area. One question mark (?) signifies that preliminary information appears positive in a limited number of studies. Two question marks (??) signify that preliminary information is limited but that a positive effect has been suggested by one or more investigators. Three question marks (???) signify that the information is very preliminary and efficacy is questionable, or a lack of efficacy has been reported.

This handbook is not intended to encourage the use of psychotropics in children or adolescents. Psychotropic drugs may be indicated when behavioral or other therapies fail, or when drug therapy allows the child or adolescent to function in a more normal manner. Due to the limited information on the use of psychotropic drugs in the pediatric population, practitioners are encouraged to use their best judgment and clinical skills in the treatment of these patients.

Acknowledgements

The author wishes to acknowledge her parents, Arllen and Victoria Theesen, and her colleagues, Dr. Jack E. Fincham, Dr. Paul M. Fine, and Dr. Glen L. Stimmel, for their encouragement.

Chapter 1

Central Nervous System Stimulants

Dextroamphetamine sulfate

Dexedrine® is marketed by SmithKline Beecham.
Dextroamphetamine is also available in generic form.

Methylphenidate hydrochloride

Ritalin® is marketed by Ciba Pharmaceuticals.
Methylphenidate is also available in generic form.

Pemoline, Magnesium

Cylert® is marketed by Abbott Laboratories.

DSM-IV INDICATIONS

Attention-Deficit/Hyperactivity Disorder (ADHD)

FDA: Approved for Attention Deficit Disorders (approved prior to DSM-IV) (*PDR*, 1994).
USP: Accepted for ADHD (*USPDI*, 1994).

CONTRAINDICATIONS: Hypersensitivity to the individual agents; cardiovascular disease, hypertension; marked anxiety, tension, agitation, or psychosis; history of drug dependence; during or within 14 days following administration of monoamine oxidase inhibitors; patients with verbal or motor tics or a family history of Tourette's syndrome (*see* ADHD and Tourette's); for the use of dextroamphetamine, hypersensitivity to related sympathomimetic amines; for the Dexedrine® products, tartrazine sensitivity; and for pemoline, hepatic insufficiency.

PHARMACOLOGY: Dextroamphetamine is the dextrorotatory isomer of amphetamine. Methylphenidate is a piperidine derivative structurally similar to the amphetamines, however pemoline is structurally dissimilar to the amphetamines. Dextroamphetamine, methylphenidate, and pemoline increase the activity of the neurotransmitters, norepinephrine and dopamine. The CNS (central nervous system) stimulants increase the release of the neurotransmitters and inhibit the reuptake of the neurotransmitters into the presynaptic neuron. The CNS stimulants also inhibit the activity of the monoamine oxidase enzyme. Methylphenidate may also have direct post-synaptic agonist activity. Each of the CNS stimulants work through a slightly different mechanism; therefore, nonresponse to one stimulant does not indicate nonresponse to another (Wilens and Biederman, 1992).

Even though the pharmacological effects of the CNS stimulants have been studied, the exact mechanism of action involved in the treatment of ADHD has not been determined. The main sites of action for the CNS stimulants appear to be the cerebral cortex, striatum (Lou et al., 1989), and possibly the reticular activating system. The reticular activating system is central to the integration of stimuli from the environment and presenting these to the cerebral cortex. The inhibitory pathways of the locus ceruleus aid in focusing attention by filtering competing stimuli. These inhibitory pathways are mediated by norepinephrine, and they reduce excessive variability in arousal and reactivity. It has been observed that the stimulants reach their maximum clinical effects during the absorption phase and not at peak blood levels. The absorption phase parallels the acute release of norepinephrine and dopamine into synaptic clefts, suggesting that the alteration of dopamine and norepinephrine activity may be the basis for stimulant drug action in ADHD (Zametkin and Borcherding, 1989). Unfortunately, the studies of urinary catecholamine metabolites in untreated children with ADHD in comparison to controls and after drug therapy are inconclusive (Zametkin and Rapoport, 1987). The studies of CNS stimulant induced effects on growth hormone and prolactin are also inconclusive, but suggest a lack of effect on hypothalamic function (Zametkin and Rapoport, 1987; Shaywitz et al., 1990).

Various models of arousal have been proposed to explain the

effects of the stimulants on ADHD. The overarousal model assumes that the child is sympathetically driven, and the response to stimulants is paradoxical, which it is not. The underarousal model assumes that the child requires stimulant drugs to reach a certain level of arousal, thereby reducing the need for external stimulation. Neither of these models address the observation that children with ADHD have rapid, unpredictable, extreme, and poorly synchronized oscillations in levels of arousal and activity. A more recent model of drug action suggests that children with ADHD have difficulty regulating arousal in response to a particular situation. Children with ADHD may have insufficient alertness during dull and repetitive tasks and overactivity at other times, resulting in poor performance. Evans, Gualtieri, and Hicks (1986) suggest that the CNS stimulants "canalize" the extreme states of arousal allowing the patient to focus. Children with ADHD, normal children, and normal adults have the same "canalizing" effect, but children with ADHD do so to the extent that they appear to be more normal (Evans, Gualtieri, and Hicks, 1986).

EFFICACY STUDIES OF THE CENTRAL NERVOUS SYSTEM STIMULANTS

Attention-Deficit/Hyperactivity Disorder (ADHD)

Central nervous system (CNS) stimulants are the drugs of choice in the treatment of ADHD. The treatment of children with ADHD with stimulants is an accepted, but controversial practice. One of the main issues is the lack of specificity of the diagnosis of ADHD (Halperin et al., 1992). Over the last five decades, since the first observation of the positive effects of CNS stimulants on children's behavior (Bradley, 1937), there have been various terminologies (minimal brain damage, minimal brain dysfunction, hyperactivity) and definitions of the "disorder." For the most part though, the main symptoms of the disorder have remained fairly consistent. The current diagnosis includes the symptoms of hyperactivity, inattention, and impulsivity. These symptoms are inappropriate for the child's developmental level and occur in different settings. The diagnosis is based on direct observation of the child, teacher's and parents' comments, and the developmental history. There is no specific test to identify a child with ADHD.

A second controversial aspect is that the positive effects of the stimulants are nonspecific. Increased attention and decreased motor activity occur in normal children and adults, as well as children with ADHD (Rapoport et al., 1980). Therefore a positive response to stimulants is not diagnostic of ADHD. In addition, children with ADHD do not have a paradoxical "calming" response to the stimulants. The reduction in motor activity is due in part to the enhanced attention and concentration. Currently, there are no specific predictors of stimulant drug response (Jacobvitz et al., 1990).

ADHD–Short-Term Efficacy of the CNS Stimulants

The goal of drug therapy is to control the target symptoms of ADHD–inattention, impulsivity, and hyperactivity. The stimulants are more effective in treating the target symptoms than placebo, nonpharmacological therapies or no treatment in short-term trials (Pelham et al., 1993; Schachar and Tannock, 1993). Approximately 75 percent of children with ADHD will respond to stimulant drug therapy (Barkley, 1977; Wilens and Biederman, 1992). When a second stimulant is tried in children who did not respond to the first, the efficacy rating increases to 96 percent (Elia et al., 1991). For children with ADHD who are matched in age and IQ, the response rate of methylphenidate is the same for either sex (Barkley et al., 1989a; Pelham et al., 1989). Numerous short-term investigations of the various effects of the CNS stimulants in children with ADHD have been conducted (Barkley, 1977; Jacobvitz et al., 1990).

There is controversy concerning the use of the CNS stimulants in children with ADHD. Appropriate use is reserved for those children who have moderate to severe hyperactivity that occurs in different environments. CNS stimulants should not be used simply because a child does not conform to the standard classroom. The goal of drug therapy is to control the symptoms of ADHD enough to allow the child to fully participate in school. Parents and teachers should not expect the child to become symptom free and should be informed that drug therapy is limited in its effects. Learning disabilities or cognitive deficits will not be improved with drug therapy, although therapy with the CNS stimulants will allow the child to be more attentive while special education is offered. In addition, the child needs a structured home and school environment to fully address the total needs of the child with ADHD (Dulcan, 1990).

The CNS stimulants improve attention and decrease distractibility and impulsivity. The CNS stimulants also reduce the motor activity level of the child with ADHD, especially when the child is expected to be physically still. Vocalizations, noise, and disruptions in the classroom are reduced to the level of nonaffected peers (Abikoff and Gittelman, 1985). The reduction in motor activity is attributed to an indirect result of increased attention and is not apparent in all environmental settings (e.g., gymnasium, playground).

The positive cognitive effects of the CNS stimulants include improved vigilance, reaction time, short-term memory, and learning of verbal and nonverbal material (Barkley, 1977). These cognitive improvements are limited to the child's own cognitive tools and strategies as specific learning disabilities are not altered. Attentional overfocusing or cognitive perservation are considered adverse effects of the stimulants. A child with attentional overfocusing has difficulty shifting attention from one task or idea to another. The ability to shift attention is required for efficient problem solving (Tannock and Schachar, 1992). The effects of the CNS stimulants on cognitive function have been investigated in numerous studies (Jacobvitz et al., 1990; Gadow, 1992a), however specific cognitive effects are variable and are presumed to be related to dose (*see* ADHD–Effects of CNS Stimulant Dosing Regimens). The effect on cognition is difficult to determine due to the varied measurements of cognitive performance utilized and the observation that a modification of the same cognitive task (Gadow, 1992a) or a repeat measurement of the task leads to a different drug effect (Tannock and Schachar, 1992). Children who are overly preoccupied with a task, are inflexible, or zombie-like require a dose reduction or discontinuation of the stimulant. Doses of the CNS stimulants should be individualized for each child.

Early reviews of academic achievement indicate that there is minimal effect of the CNS stimulants for children with ADHD (Barkley, 1977; Gadow, 1983). Subsequent reports indicate that methylphenidate has a significant short-term effect on academic productivity and accuracy (DuPaul and Rapport, 1993; Famularo and Fenton, 1987; Pelham et al., 1985; Rapport et al., 1989). Although the effects are variable, children show an increase in the number of completed school assignments and decreased errors. As stated previously, primary learning disabilities will not be improved with the CNS stimulants.

There are multiple effects of the stimulants on interpersonal relationships. Children respond with improved compliance to adult commands and decreased oppositionality and aggression (Hinshaw, 1991; Kaplan et al., 1990). There are reciprocal improvements in the behavior of parents and caretakers during the effects of the medication. The mothers of these children respond with a decrease in commands and control over compliance and an increase in their level of non-directive interactions (Barkley, 1989b). Mothers of these children have also been reported to show increased warmth, decreased maternal criticism, and increased maternal contact (Schachar et al., 1987). The effect on peer relationships is less positive (Cunningham, Siegel, and Offord, 1985). Peers will notice an improvement in the child with ADHD who is treated with CNS stimulants, but rarely to the level of nonhyperactive peers (Whalen et al., 1989). In addition, the peers of a treated child become less aggressive and demonstrate less controlling behavior (Gadow et al., 1990a; Gadow et al., 1992b). The medications are not effective for anti-social behavior. Satterfield et al. (1994) reported that children with a high level of defiance have an increased chance of adolescent anti-social behavior, but children with ADHD and the absence of defiance are more likely than normal children to be at risk of adolescent anti-social behavior. Overall, there is an improvement in social functioning, but not normalization. The duration of action of the CNS stimulants needs to be considered when assessing the effects of the medication on peers and family members.

In general, it is recommended that the stimulants not be used in preschool children with ADHD. If parent training and a structured preschool are unsuccessful, then medication may be indicated (Speltz et al., 1988). Earlier studies (Conners, 1975; Schleifer et al., 1975) suggested that the stimulants were effective in treating preschoolers with ADHD, but were associated with impaired socialization and depression. More recent preliminary information indicates that preschoolers treated with 0.5 mg/kg of methylphenidate administered two times a day, have decreased off-task behavior and increased rates of compliance. In addition, the preschooler's duration of sustained compliance with maternal commands is increased (Barkley et al., 1984; Barkley, 1988). Few side effects were reported in these studies, however further investigations are needed, especially in a population that may not be able to describe an adverse effect. The use of stimulants in this population is very limited and requires further evaluation.

Recent investigations indicate that symptoms of ADHD extend into adolescence and adulthood (Mannuzza et al., 1993). Several short-term studies suggest that methylphenidate in doses up to 40 mg per day is just as effective for adolescents with ADHD as for children (Coons, Klorman, and Borgstedt, 1987; Evans and Pelham, 1991; Klorman, Coons, and Borgstedt, 1987; Klorman et al., 1990; Varley, 1983). Adolescents have a positive response to the stimulants with increased attention and decreased hyperactivity and oppositionality. Overall, in comparison to the studies in children, there are few studies of adolescents with ADHD (Greenhill and Setterberg, 1993). Resistance to utilize the stimulants in the adolescent population is attributed to three concerns. First, the inaccurate "paradoxical" calming effect of the stimulants for children was believed to change at puberty resulting in a more "normal" response. This concern is inaccurate, and studies have demonstrated that the effect of the stimulants is similar for children, adolescents, and adults with ADHD. The second concern is substance abuse by the adolescent. Although investigations have indicated that adolescents who were treated with stimulants as children are not more likely than their peers to abuse substances, follow-up studies of treated adolescents are indicated to fully evaluate this issue. The third concern is growth suppression and other adverse effects. Adolescence is a period of rapid growth, and whether or not the stimulants effect growth has not been evaluated (Varley, 1985). Further investigations of dose response, adverse effects, and multimodal therapy (Brown, Borden, and Clingerman, 1985a) are indicated for adolescents with ADHD.

ADHD–Effects of CNS Stimulant Dosing Regimens

Currently, it is recommended that the dosing of CNS stimulants be individualized according to response. The difficulty with this recommendation is deciding how to measure response and which response to measure (Barkley, 1977; Gadow, 1992a; Jacobvitz et al., 1990). It has been suggested that the CNS stimulants have different effects at different doses. An initial study by Sprague and Sleator (1977) reported on the dose-response effects of methylphenidate. They reported that for cognitive tasks that were quite easy, there was no difference between placebo, methylphenidate 0.3 mg/kg, and methylphenidate 1.0 mg/kg. For difficult cognitive tasks they found a different pattern. They observed that improvement peaks for difficult cognitive tasks at morning doses of methylphenidate 0.3 mg/kg, but a reduction of cognitive ability is observed at higher doses of methylphenidate 1.0 mg/kg. Teacher ratings and motor activity improved with increasing dose, with maximum improvement at a dose of 1.0 mg/kg. The authors suggest that different doses can have different effects on target behaviors and that titrating the dose to social behavior may not be optimal for learning.

Subsequent reports using a wide variety of measures of cognitive performance support, extend, or refute the findings of Sprague and Sleator (1977). The studies indicate that there are complex and varying effects of increasing dose levels, which may be beneficial for one target system (e.g., behavior) and adverse in terms of another system (e.g., cognitive or social functioning). In addition, it appears that these effects may be independent of dose for a specific child. Therefore, it is important to determine the dose response for an individual child based on numerous sources (parents and teachers), and adjust the dose and schedule to obtain the maximum overall response, with minimal adverse effects.

Behavioral rebound is a phenomenon that may occur at the end of the dosing period and is associated with the loss of CNS stimulant effect. Late in the afternoon, irritability, increased talkativeness, noncompliance, motor hyperactivity, and insomnia are signs of behavioral rebound. Behavioral rebound can be managed by administering a dose of the medication after school or combining the long and short-acting dosage forms. In some cases, adjunctive or alternative treatment such as clonidine or anti-depressants are indicated (Wilens and Biederman, 1992).

Whether or not patients develop tolerance to the CNS stimulants is not fully resolved. Noncompliance with the treatment regimen should be assessed first. There are anecdotal reports that the extended release methylphenidate may be more likely to be associated with the development of tolerance. The sustained methylphenidate blood levels may result in tolerance, tachyphylaxis, hepatic enzyme induction, or changes in receptor pharmacodynamics (Birmaher et al., 1989). The cases of 108 hyperactive children who were treated with methylphenidate over three to ten years were reviewed by Safer and Allen (1989). They reported that the dose of methylphenidate, when adjusted for growth, did not change significantly during the three to ten years of treatment. In addition, the commonly used milligram per kilogram dose overcorrected for growth as the child aged. This suggests that a slightly lower total daily dose than the calculated milligram per kilogram dose can be used for older children. In this study, a loss of previously satisfactory response was uncommon (6 percent) and was associated with noncompliance and lower than standard doses. In this retrospective review, three of the 108 children were assessed to have developed tolerance to the effects of methylphenidate.

ADHD–Long-Term Efficacy of the CNS Stimulants

In comparison to the short-term effects, the long-term risks and benefits of the CNS stimulants are less clear. The long-term studies of the use of CNS stimulants have been extensively analyzed and criticized. Part of the discussion is the more recent observation that many children do not grow out of the disorder. In addition, children with ADHD are not a homogeneous group and present with other disorders including anxiety, depression, oppositional/conduct disorder, Tourette's disorder, and learning disabilities (Biederman, Newcorn, and Sprich, 1991). This comorbidity affects the outcome of the long-term studies. Subgroups of patients may respond differently to a treatment regimen or have different risk factors, and only recently have these subgroups of patients been identified by researchers (Biederman, Newcorn, and Sprich, 1991).

The currently available long-term studies of children with ADHD suggest little long-term impact of stimulant drugs on scholastic achievement, peer relationships, or behavior problems in adolescence (Gadow, 1983; Hechtman, 1985; Jacobvitz et al., 1990; Klein and Mannuzza, 1991; Mannuzza et al., 1993; Satterfield et al., 1994). However, these studies are controversial for many reasons. First, most of the studies assessed adolescents or adults who were treated with CNS stimulants as children. These children were not randomly assigned to different treatment groups over time, and these studies, like many long-term studies, most likely included participants who are more severely affected. Second, the long-term studies do not include a placebo-control group. Although, due to the impressive short-term effects of the CNS stimulants, randomization to placebo for a long-term study may be unethical. Third, the lack of recognition of the diagnostic heterogeneity of the ADHD disorder and the comorbidity with ADHD decreases the homogeneity of the participants in long-term studies. Fourth, CNS stimulant doses were adjusted in a clinical setting and may not have been at the optimal dose or may have not been given for a long enough period of time. Fifth, the effects of the CNS stimulants are limited and will not change long-term cognitive deficits or learning disabilities. Sixth, noncompliance with a treatment regimen occurs frequently in the pediatric population (Brown, Borden, and Clingerman, 1985b), and many of the long-term studies did not address this issue. Finally, the CNS stimulants are unlikely to change a child's low self-esteem, social skills deficit, or family pathology (Schachar, 1993). Although the perfect long-term study will probably not be conducted, it is necessary to prospectively address some of the issues above in order to more accurately determine the long-term effect of these medications.

Comorbidity with ADHD

More recently published studies have acknowledged that hyperactive children who are referred for psychiatric evaluation (and subsequently participate in psychopharmacological research) are a heterogeneous population (Gadow, 1992a). These children present with varying symptoms of ADHD and with comorbid disorders such as conduct or oppositional disorder, mood disorders, anxiety disorders, learning disabilities, mental retardation, Tourette's syndrome, and borderline personality disorder (Biederman, 1991). How comorbidity will effect drug therapy or how drug therapy will effect comorbidity has only recently been investigated.

ADHD and Anxiety/Depression

The treatment of ADHD and anxiety/depression has recently been investigated. Pliszka (1989) reports that children with ADHD and comorbid anxiety showed less impulsiveness and increased reaction times in comparison to children with ADHD and without anxiety. In addition, children with ADHD and comorbid anxiety had a decreased response to the stimulants than those children without anxiety, while the comorbidity of oppositionality or conduct disorder did not affect stimulant response. In contrast, Livingston, Dykman, and Ackerman (1992) report that there is no evidence that children with ADHD and comorbid anxiety or depression, oppositionality, or conduct disorder respond any less well to a CNS stimulant than children with ADHD and without comorbidity. These preliminary investigations require replication in order to determine the effects of the comorbidity on the efficacy of the CNS stimulants.

ADHD and Autism

Autism in manifested with the symptoms of stereotypic behaviors, lability of mood, and pervasive impairment in social, cognitive, and communication development. In addition the target symptoms of impulsiveness, short attention span, and hyperactivity are observed in patients with autism. In the past, the use of the CNS stimulants in patients with autism was contraindicated. Recently, the case studies of nine children with autism suggest that methylphenidate may be effective in reducing the target symptoms of hyperactivity and inattention (Birmaher, Quintana, and Greenhill, 1988). Methylphenidate administered in doses between 10 to 50 mg per day for two weeks did not worsen the stereotypic movements or induce psychotic symptoms in this group of patients. A second case report of a six-year-old autistic boy that used a placebo-control suggests that methylphenidate 0.5 mg/kg improves attention, hyperactivity, destructive behavior, and stereotyped movements (Strayhorn et al., 1988). In this case report, unhappiness and tantrums increased with the use of methylphenidate. These preliminary results indicate further investigations are warranted.

ADHD and Fragile X Syndrome

Hagerman, Murphy, and Wittenberger (1988) studied 15 children with the Fragile X Syndrome and attentional problems. The patients had a mean IQ score of 58. Patients were randomly assigned to placebo, dextroamphetamine, or methylphenidate in a double-blind, crossover design. Each drug phase was conducted for seven days. The doses of methylphenidate used were 0.3 mg/kg administered twice a day. The dose of dextroamphetamine was 0.2 mg/kg administered once per day in the extended release form. Both stimulants improved behaviors, although for most measures only methylphenidate was statistically significant. The substantial difference between the doses of the methylphenidate and the dextroamphetamine may account for the decreased effect of the dextroamphetamine (Hagerman, Murphy, and Wittenberger, 1988). This is a very preliminary report and further studies are needed.

ADHD and Mental Retardation

Biederman, Newcorn, and Sprich (1991) report that ADHD is three to four times more prevalent in children with mental retardation than children with normal IQ. Case studies suggest that the CNS stimulants are effective in reducing hyperactivity and aggression, and increasing on-task behavior in children with ADHD and mental retardation. These case studies also suggest that the response to the CNS stimulants is more variable in this population and can be associated with decreased levels of social interaction and dose-related dyskinetic movements (Payton et al., 1989; Gadow, Pomeroy, and Nolan, 1992c). Two double-blind, crossover, placebo-controlled studies indicate that higher functioning children with ADHD and mental retardation have a more positive response to methylphenidate. In contrast, lower functioning children are less likely to show a positive response and are more susceptible to adverse effects (Aman et al., 1991a; Aman et al., 1991b; Handen et al., 1992).

There was no reported effect on learning. The adverse effects consisted of severe social withdrawal and appearance of motor tics (Handen et al., 1991). These preliminary studies indicate that there is a greater variability in response to the CNS stimulants in this population, and that cautious monitoring of drug effect is necessary.

ADHD and Tourette's Syndrome

Between 35 percent and 70 percent of children who develop Tourette's syndrome have symptoms of ADHD. The symptoms of ADHD are observed up to 2.5 years prior to the onset of the Tourette's syndrome (Gadow and Sverd, 1990b). The CNS stimulants are the drugs of choice to treat ADHD, however they may be associated with the onset or exacerbation of tics. In the past, the use of the CNS stimulants was contraindicated in children who had Tourette's syndrome or had a family history of tics or Tourette's syndrome (Lowe et al., 1982). Recent studies (Erenberg, Cruse, and Rothner, 1985) have indicated that the CNS stimulants have a variable effect on the frequency of tics. The use of the CNS stimulants is associated with an increase, decrease, and no change on the frequency of tics. For a patient with Tourette's syndrome, this observation may be due to the waxing and waning of the symptoms of Tourette's syndrome and not to drug therapy (Gadow and Sverd, 1990b).

Part of the controversy of this issue is the question, what is considered to be a high dose of the CNS stimulants? Investigators (Gadow, Nolan, and Sverd, 1992d) have shown that methylphenidate in the range of 0.1 mg/kg to 0.5 mg/kg is not associated with an exacerbation of tics, but effectively suppressed the symptoms of hyperactivity, which is the primary complaint of care givers. Higher doses of methylphenidate may or may not show a different effect. The controversy of how to treat a child with ADHD and Tourette's continues when the practitioner considers the issue of relative risk (Gadow and Sverd, 1990b). Gadow and Sverd (1990b) point out that all of the commonly prescribed drugs for ADHD and Tourette's (CNS stimulants, neuroleptics, tricyclic antidepressants, and clonidine) are associated with the induction or exacerbation of tics. In addition, each of the drugs used carries comparable risk of other adverse effects.

Drug Holidays

A drug holiday consists of a trial period off medication and is used to determine the need for continued medication therapy. The duration of the holiday and when it should be conducted during the school year varies according to the patient and is at the discretion of the practitioner. Summer drug holidays are used to avoid interfering with school performance. Some practitioners advocate for drug holidays at the beginning of the school year to see if a new teacher and classroom make a difference. Others suggest avoiding drug holidays at the beginning of the year to avoid "labeling" of the child in the early part of the school year by the teacher or classmates. In addition, if children do poorly in the first few months of school, they become frustrated in their effort to make up for lost time, low grades, and poor impressions (Dulcan, 1990). Annual drug holidays are necessary to prevent growth suppression (*see* Adverse Effects–growth suppression). If the child is on a high daily dose or has significant afternoon rebound, tapering of the dose is recommended to avoid further rebound effects (Dulcan, 1990).

Medication Placebo Trial

A medication placebo trial may be helpful for objectively determining the positive and negative effects of the CNS stimulants (Fine and Jewesson, 1989; McBride, 1988). Placebo trials may be useful when the child, parent, or teacher are overly enthusiastic or overly negative about medications. During a placebo trial, the patient, parent, and teacher are "blinded" to the order of the drug/placebo administration. The physician may decide to be "blinded" as well. The pharmacist prepares identical gelatin capsules containing either the medication or placebo. A schedule is prepared for drug/placebo administration for the patient. Different doses of medication and different dosing regimens can be used depending upon the clinical questions that need answered. Parents and teachers are asked to fill out rating forms for positive effects and side effects in each condition.

After completion of the trial, the rating scales are scored and comparisons are made with the schedule of medication/placebo administered. Potentially, by determining the effects of the medications, parents and teachers will become more objective in their viewpoint. Fine and Jewesson (1989) point out that there are several problems in administering a medication placebo trial. Even though capsules were dispensed in clearly marked envelopes for each day, parents claimed to have been confused about the correct envelope for the day. Parents and teachers also forgot to fill in the rating forms. Some teachers declined to participate because of their objections to giving children medication to change their behavior. Fine and Jewesson suggest that compliance with the therapeutic regimen be assessed before determining the efficacy or side effects of the medication.

Multimodal Therapy

After the initial long-term studies indicated that drug therapy was not effective in modifying the outcome of the child with ADHD, multimodal therapy was suggested (Barkley, 1977). Multimodal therapy combines two or more therapies (drug therapy, family therapy, special education, behavioral modification, and individual psychotherapy) to treat the child. Multimodal therapy is more likely to address the heterogeneity of the individual child. The few studies that have been conducted indicate that there is minimal effect of multimodal therapy on long-term outcome (Horn et al., 1991; Ialongo, Horn, and Pascoe, 1993; Satterfield et al., 1994); however more extensive research is needed. Practitioners are encouraged to remain motivated to treat the child in a comprehensive manner and not just to medicate.

Efficacy of Drug Combinations

For most children a stimulant medication is all that will be required to effectively treat ADHD. If the first stimulant tried is not effective, an alternate stimulant is indicated. Up to 96 percent of children were effectively treated with one or another stimulant in a study by Elia et al. (1991). Alternative therapies are indicated when stimulants are contraindicated, there is an inadequate response to stimulants, or more commonly if adverse effects such as anorexia or insomnia prevent an adequate response. Alternative therapies include tricyclic antidepressants, bupropion, or clonidine. Combinations of drugs (e.g., methylphenidate and a tricyclic antidepressant, or methylphenidate and clonidine) may be indicated after several individual drug therapies have failed or when the patient presents with comorbidity (e.g., ADHD and Tourette's).

DEVELOPMENTAL PHARMACOKINETICS

Dextroamphetamine

Absorption: Absorption is rapid, with large variations in the peak plasma levels.

Onset of action: Effects may be observed within 30 to 60 minutes.

Time to peak effect/peak plasma levels: Peak plasma levels and peak effect occur in three to four hours. There is a large variation (up to 30-fold) in peak plasma levels for the standard release formulation (Brown et al., 1979). The variation in peak plasma level for the extended release formulation is up to 3 fold (Brown et al., 1980).

Duration of action: Duration of activity of dextroamphetamine in any dosage form is usually not greater than four hours (Brown et al., 1980). The extended release dosage form may have a duration of activity of two to nine hours (Pelham et al., 1990).

Half-life: In children, the half-life is 6.6 to 8.4 hours (Brown et al., 1980).

Plasma levels: The effects of dextroamphetamine appear to be related to the rapid absorption phase and are not correlated to specific peak or trough plasma levels. Plasma levels are not clinically useful at this time.

Methylphenidate

Absorption: There is rapid absorption from the standard release product. The rate of absorption may be increased if taken with food, however the amount absorbed remains constant whether given with food or not (Chan et al., 1983). The clinical effects of methylphenidate are not modified when administered with food (Swanson et al., 1983). The absorption from the extended release product is slower.

Bioavailability: The bioavailability varies from 10.5 to 52.4 percent (Chan et al., 1983).

Distribution: Protein binding is 15 percent. Methylphenidate rapidly crosses the blood-brain barrier.

Onset of action: 30 to 60 minutes for the standard release product, and one to two hours for the extended release product (Pelham et al., 1987).

Time to peak effect/peak plasma levels: One to two hours for the standard release product (Gualtieri et al., 1982; Shaywitz, Hunt, and Jatlow, 1982). Two to five hours after the extended release product (Birmaher et al., 1989).

Duration of action: Duration of action is four to six hours for the standard release product and two to nine hours for the extended release product (Pelham et al., 1990).

Half-life: The half-life of methylphenidate in children is two to four hours (Gualtieri et al., 1982; Shaywitz, Hunt, and Jatlow, 1982).

Plasma/salivary levels: There is interindividual and, in some cases, intraindividual variation in plasma levels per dose (Gualtieri et al., 1982). Plasma levels are not clinically useful at this time. Saliva concentrations of methylphenidate are not independent of salivary flow, and therefore are not accurate indicators of methylphenidate plasma levels (Greenhill et al., 1987).

Pemoline, Magnesium

Absorption: The absorption of pemoline is slow and erratic.

Bioavailability: Pemoline exhibits a wide variation (up to 200 percent) in bioavailability (Sallee et al., 1985).

Distribution: In adults, protein binding is less than 40 percent.

Onset of action: At higher doses (2mg/kg), the onset of action can be at two hours (Sallee, Stiller, and Perel, 1992), but the incidence of adverse effects increases (*see* Adverse Effects–abnormal involuntary movements). Lower initial doses with subsequent titration may require up to three weeks to see full effect.

Time to peak effect/peak plasma levels: Pemoline peak plasma levels occur in one to 5.5 hours (Sallee et al., 1985).

Duration of action: The effects of pemoline may last six to nine hours (Sallee, Stiller, and Perel, 1992; Pelham et al., 1990).

Half-life: For a single dose of pemoline, the half-life varies from 2.1 to 12.4 hours with a mean of 7.28 to 8.6 hours (Sallee et al., 1985; Collier et al., 1985). In children, the half-life increases with age, up to the adult half-life of 12 hours (Collier et al., 1985).

Plasma levels: A wide variation has been found in pemoline serum levels. Sallee, Stiller, and Perel (1992) suggest that it is unlikely that pemoline accumulates in the body and that intersubject variability in response may be due to variability in bioavailability. Plasma levels do not appear to be clinically helpful at this time.

DOSAGE RANGES

Attention Deficit Hyperactivity Disorder (*See also*, ADHD–Effects of CNS Stimulant Dosing Regimens)

Although dosage guidelines include a milligram per kilogram dose, individual response is idiosyncratic and does not appear to be related to body weight (Rapport, DuPaul, and Kelly, 1989). The dosing of CNS stimulants should be individualized according to response and adverse effects. The dosing schedule should be modified to fit the individual needs of the child and family. The short and long-acting preparations can be used to maximize positive effects and minimize adverse effects. Children may take medication during the week only, while others require dosing after school and/or on weekends. Drug holidays are recommended during the school year and during summer vacations to assess drug efficacy and to allow for growth of the child. There are dosage guidelines for children three to five years of age for dextroamphetamine; however medication is usually administered after parent training and a structured preschool environment are unsuccessful. In addition, adverse effects may occur more frequently in the preschool population (Barkley, 1988). Most children begin CNS stimulant therapy after beginning regular school.

Dextroamphetamine: For children, three to five years of age, the initial dose is 2.5 mg. The dose is increased by 2.5 mg/day at weekly intervals. The usual dosing range is 0.1 to 0.5 mg/kg/day. The extended release forms of dextroamphetamine are not indicated for children less than six years.

For children six years and older, the initial dose is 5 mg once or twice daily with increases of 5 mg/day at weekly intervals. The usual dosing range is 0.1 to 0.5 mg/kg/day. The maximum daily dose is 40 mg per day (*see also* ADHD–Effects of CNS Stimulant Dosing Regimens). The extended release products may be used on a once a day basis. The standard release products are given in the morning and at noon.

Methylphenidate: For children six years and older, the initial dose is 5 mg once or twice a day. Doses less than 5 mg are not recommended. The 5 mg tablet is not scored and is not easily breakable. The maximum daily dose is 60 mg (*see also* ADHD–Effects of CNS Stimulant Dosing Regimens). The extended release form of methylphenidate may be substituted for the regular dosage form in a corresponding total daily dose. The use of the extended release product may be beneficial for a child that does not want to take the medication at lunch or when the school system will not allow administration of the drug at school. Although there were initial reports of decreased efficacy of the extended release product in comparison to the standard product (Pelham et al., 1987), subsequent studies have reported no significant difference in efficacy between products (Pelham et al., 1990; Fitzpatrick et al., 1992). The authors note that individual response varies with different dosing regimens. The extended release tablets have a reported duration of action of two to nine hours (*see* methylphenidate pharmacokinetics) and have been combined with the standard release product (Fitzpatrick et al., 1992). In order to maintain the wax matrix and the controlled release of methylphenidate, the extended release product, Ritalin SR®, is to be swallowed whole and not chewed (Rosse and Licamele, 1984).

Pemoline, Magnesium: For children six years and older, the initial dose is 37.5 mg once daily in the morning. The dose is increased by 18.75 mg/day on a weekly basis according to response. Some children may need twice daily doses. The maximum recommended dose is 112.5 mg/day.

ADVERSE EFFECTS REPORTED IN CHILDREN AND ADOLESCENTS

COMMON

Prior to the initiation of drug therapy a baseline assessment of the child's common complaints should be obtained. This assessment can be helpful later in determining whether or not the child is developing an adverse effect to the drug. The management of side effects includes monitoring for continued effect, decreasing the dose, discontinuation, or trying a different CNS stimulant.

Anorexia: Patients should be monitored for changes in appetite or dietary habits. Baseline assessments of eating habits suggest that children with ADHD are picky eaters, even before CNS stimulants (Dulcan, 1990). Administering the medication after the meal may decrease the anorexia. A high-calorie late evening snack may be helpful.

Insomnia: Difficulty getting to sleep is a frequent adverse effect (Ahmann et al., 1993; Barkley et al., 1990; Fine and Johnston, 1993). The short-acting products are less likely than the extended release products to affect sleep. Whether pemoline is more likely to be associated with insomnia due to the longer half-life is unknown. Dosage and schedule adjustments may be helpful in alleviating this adverse effect by administering the last dose of the day at 4 p.m. Sedative-hypnotics are generally not indicated. In a case report of a nine-year-old boy, Rubenstein, Silver, and Licamele (1994) described the use of clonidine 0.05 mg at bedtime to treat stimulant-induced insomnia.

Gastrointestinal upset: Abdominal pain or stomachaches occur frequently in this population prior to drug therapy. Stomachaches that are associated with drug therapy can be minimized by administering with food or reducing the dose.

Growth suppression: The CNS stimulants are associated with significant growth suppression; however, the long-term growth effects appear to be minimal (Dickinson et al., 1979; Friedman et al., 1981; Gross, 1976; Klein et al., 1988a; Satterfield et al., 1979). Children during the first year of therapy have significant growth suppression that is followed by growth acceleration during the second year. Drug holidays are associated with growth rebound (Klein and Mannuzza, 1988b). Height and weight growth suppression may be more likely in children who are receiving high doses of CNS stimulants or in a subpopulation of children with ADHD (Mattes and Gittleman, 1983). Dextroamphetamine may be more likely than methylphenidate to be associated with height and weight growth suppression (Safer, Allen, and Barr, 1972). This difference may be due to the longer half-life of dextroamphetamine (Greenhill, Puig-Antich, and Novacenko, 1984). Most of the long-term studies of growth suppression have studied adolescents or adults who were treated with CNS stimulants as children (Klein et al., 1988a). A preliminary chart review of 31 adolescents indicates that treatment with methylphenidate (0.75 mg/kg/day) does not affect adolescent growth velocities over a 6- to 12-month period (Vincent, Varley, and Leger, 1990). The consequences of longer treatment or higher doses during adolescence into adulthood are unknown. CNS stimulant-induced growth suppression remains a controversial area. Monitoring of height and weight is necessary.

LESS COMMON

Drowsiness, dizziness, nausea, euphoria, nightmares, tremor, dry mouth, constipation, and lethargy (Barkley, 1977) may occur during treatment. Depression may occur during treatment or upon withdrawal (Brown and Sexson, 1988). For these side effects, dosage reduction or discontinuation is indicated.

Central Nervous System: Headaches, anxiousness, dysphoria, irritability, and social withdrawal may occur. There can be a high rate of irritability, anxiousness, dysphoria, and proneness to crying prior to the use of the CNS stimulants, therefore a baseline comparison should be made (Ahmann et al., 1993; Barkley et al., 1990). In general, these side effects require dosage reduction or discontinuation.

Behavioral rebound: This phenomenon occurs at the end of the dosing period (after school) and is associated with the shorter acting preparations. The frequency of this effect is controversial (Wilens and Biederman, 1992) and has been reported as a rare effect and not clinically significant (Johnston et al., 1988). This particular side effect can be very upsetting to parents and is commonly confused with the return of symptoms (*see* ADHD–Effects of CNS Stimulant Dosing Regimens).

Tics: The use of the CNS stimulants is associated with the onset, the exacerbation, or a reduction in the frequency of tics (Erenberg, Cruse, and Rothner, 1985). The use of the CNS stimulants may be associated with the earlier onset of Tourette's syndrome (Golden, 1988) in a susceptible child. If tics develop while a child is taking a CNS stimulant, the drug should be discontinued and the child reassessed. Non-drug techniques should be employed, and the use of drugs should be avoided if possible (*see* ADHD and Tourette's syndrome).

Hepatotoxicity: Pemoline has been associated with elevated transaminases, alkaline phosphatase, LDH and bilirubin, hepatotoxicity, and liver failure. Routine liver function tests are indicated every two weeks for the first six weeks during dose titration and then every two to three months, or as clinical symptoms (fatigue, nausea, and vomiting) warrant during therapy (Pratt and Dubois, 1990; Patterson, 1984).

Cardiovascular: In children with ADHD, methylphenidate is associated with minor increases (11 beats/minute) in heart rate during the initial dosing period. Methylphenidate is associated with statistically significant increase in blood pressure but this effect is not considered to be clinically important (Safer, 1992). An exception to this finding is that diastolic blood pressure may be increased in black adolescents (Brown and Sexson, 1989). The effects of methylphenidate on the EKG are limited, and significant conduction abnormalities are usually not found. Amphetamine and pemoline have not been reported to cause clinically significant increases in heart rate or blood pressure, although neither drug has been evaluated as well as methylphenidate. EKG effects have not been investigated in children taking dextroamphetamine or pemoline (Safer, 1992). Most investigations used moderate doses of methylphenidate (20 to 30 mg per day), dextroamphetamine (10 to 25 mg per day), or pemoline (70 mg per day). Higher doses may be associated with an increased frequency of cardiovascular adverse effects.

Abnormal involuntary movements: In high doses, the CNS stimulants are associated with the induction of abnormal involuntary movements (Sallee et al, 1989; Gay and Ryan, 1994). Sallee et al. (1985) reported that initial doses of pemoline 2 mg/kg resulted in a faster onset of action. Sallee et al. (1989) subsequently reported that the same dose resulted in several children developing abnormal involuntary movements within two to three hours. These movements consisted of buccal-lingual chewing movements; choreoathetoid movements of the trunk, leg, finger, or jaw; cheek puffing; lip smacking; eye blinking; and ballistic movements. The half-life and peak plasma levels of pemoline did not differ between the children who developed the abnormal involuntary movements and the children who did not. Lower initial and total doses may avoid this complication.

Psychosis: Stereotyped movements, delusions, disjointed thinking, visual and tactile hallucinations have been reported at low and high doses. Mania has also been reported (Koehler-Troy, Strober, and Malenbaum, 1986). Discontinuation of the stimulant is necessary (Barkley, 1977; Bloom et al., 1988; Licamele, 1988; Lucas and Weiss, 1971).

Alopecia: Only one case report of alopecia was found (Lucas and Weiss, 1971).

Leukocytosis: A decrease in white blood cells is listed in the product information for methylphenidate, but is not reported in clinical studies (Wilens and Biederman, 1992). An annual routine physical exam should include a complete blood count.

Seizures: Methylphenidate 0.6 mg/kg/day is not associated with an increase in seizure frequency in children stabilized on anti-convulsant medications (Crumrine et al., 1987; Feldman et al., 1989; McBride, Wang, and Torres, 1986).

Angina, arrhythmia's: These cardiovascular effects are listed in the product information, but are not reported in clinical studies of children with ADHD (Safer, 1992).

ALLERGIC REACTION: Products (e.g., Dexedrine®) that contain FD&C Yellow No. 5 (tartrazine) may cause an allergic-type reaction in susceptible individuals. Tartrazine sensitivity is frequently seen in patients who also have aspirin hypersensitivity. The hypersensitivity reactions to methylphenidate may include skin rash, urticaria, fever, arthralgia, exfoliative dermatitis, and erythema multiform.

TOXICITY: Signs and symptoms of toxicity include supranormalization (Gadow, 1992a), overfocusing, extreme quietness, socially withdrawing, decline in school work (Dulcan, 1990), agitation, confusion, convulsions, delirium, hallucinations, false sense of well-being, hyperpyrexia, tachycardia, fever, sweating, increased blood pressure, muscle twitching, trembling or tremors, and vomiting.

DRUG INTERACTIONS

DRUG	DRUGS	EFFECT
CNS Stimulants*	Tricyclic antidepressants	Concurrent use may increase cardiovascular effects, possibly resulting in arrhythmias, tachycardia, or severe hypertension or hyperpyrexia. (See Methylphenidate below.) Monitoring is recommended.
CNS Stimulants*	Insulin, antidiabetic agents	Concurrent use may increase hyperglycemia.
CNS Stimulants*	Anti-hypertensive agents	Loss of anti-hypertensive effect may occur; monitoring is suggested.
CNS Stimulants*	Digoxin, Levodopa	Increased risk of cardiac arrhthymia.
CNS Stimulants*	Anti-psychotic agents, e.g., haloperidol, loxapine, molindone, phenothiazines, pimozide, thioxanthenes	Concurrent use may reduce the effect of either agent and is usually contraindicated in the treatment of ADHD (Gualtieri and Hicks, 1985).
CNS Stimulants*	Lithium	Lithium may reduce the effects of the CNS stimulants.
CNS Stimulants*	Meperidine, Monoamine oxidase inhibitors	Concurrent use is not recommended and may result in severe hypertensive and hyperpyretic

		crisis, with headache, cardiac arrhythmias, vomiting, respiratory depression, convulsions, coma, vascular collapse, and death. CNS stimulants should not be administered within 14 days of a MAO-I or meperidine.
CNS Stimulants*	CNS stimulants, e.g., local anesthetics, appetite suppressants, bupropion, caffeine, cocaine, fluoxetine, sertraline, sympathomimetics, theophylline and derivatives, etc.	Concurrent use may result in additive CNS stimulation resulting in excessive nervousness, irritability, insomnia, possible seizures, or cardiac arrhythmias.
Dextroamphetamine	Acidifiers, e.g., ascorbic acid, fruit juices, etc.	Concurrent use may decrease the effects of dextroamphetamine by increasing urinary elimination. Excessive amounts of acidifers are required to decrease urine pH.
	Alkalizers, e.g., calcium or magnesium containing antacids, etc.	Concurrent use may increase the effects of dextroamphetamine by decreasing urinary elimination. Excessive amounts of alkalizers are required to increase pH.
Dextroamphetamine	Ethosuximide, phenobarbital, phenytoin	Concurrent use may delay the intestinal absorption of the anticonvulsants, requiring dosage adjustments.
Methylphenidate	Anticoagulants (coumarin), anti-convulsants (phenobarbital, phenytoin, primidone), tricyclic antidepressants, fluoxetine	Methylphenidate may inhibit the metabolism of these drugs, thereby increasing the blood levels or pharmacological effect. A dosage reduction may be necessary. The combination of methylphenidate and imipramine has resulted in confusion, marked agression and severe agitation, even psychosis

(Grob and Coyle, 1986), although this combination has been
used successfully.

Pemoline   Anti-convulsants   Pemoline may reduce the seizure
threshold; therefore, dosage ad-
justments of the anti-convulsants
may be necessary.

*CNS Stimulants include dextroamphetamine, methylphenidate, and magne-
sium pemoline.

MONITORING GUIDELINES

Baseline Assessment:

- Obtain baseline rating scales, such as the Conners Abbre-
viated Teacher Rating Scales and the Conners Parent
Questionnaires (Conners and Barkley, 1985), to determine
pre-drug symptomatology. Other rating scales are also uti-
lized (Greenhill, 1992)
- History and physical, including height and weight of the
patient.
- Blood pressure and pulse.
- Observe for involuntary movements, tics.
- Determine the family or individual history for tic disorder or
Tourette's syndrome. If positive, determine the risk: benefit
ratio for the possibility of the stimulants inducing tics.
- For pemoline, baseline liver function tests, including ALT
(Alanine aminotransferase), AST (Aspartate aminotrans-
ferase), LDH (Lactate dehydrogenase).
- Other laboratory tests as indicated.
- Baseline history of physical complaints, and sleeping and
eating habits.

Time Pattern for Response:

- The CNS stimulants have a rapid onset of action and effects can be observed after the first dose. Care givers
should administer the medication after or during meals to

minimize the reduction in appetite. Rarely, tolerance to the effects of the CNS stimulants has been observed. It is controversial whether tolerance is due to decreased drug response, noncompliance, or other factors.

Follow-Up Assessment:

- Rating scales and reports from teachers and parents on the effectiveness of the medication should be obtained during the dose titration period. A 20 percent reduction in the rating scale score indicates a positive response (Greenhill, 1992), but overall assessment is made on an individual basis.
- Height and weight should be followed every three months and compared to standard growth charts. For weight reduction or lack of weight gain, administer the medications after meals. For height growth reduction use the lowest effective dose and drug holidays.
- Blood pressure and pulse should routinely be obtained during dose titration and during follow-up; however, minimal changes, if any, are usually observed in cardiovascular healthy patients (Safer, 1992). Patients with cardiovascular abnormalities may require more extensive monitoring.
- Titration of the dosage and modification of the dosing schedule according to the individual patient are considered hallmarks of appropriate prescribing.
- Monitor appetite changes and sleep patterns.
- Monitor for motor and vocal tics, and other involuntary movements.
- Complete blood cell tests with differential and platelet counts are recommended on an annual basis or as indicated by patient status for patients on prolonged methylphenidate therapy.
- For pemoline, monitor for early signs of hepatic insufficiency, fatigue, nausea, and vomiting. Liver functions tests (ALT, AST, and LDH) should be obtained every three to six months.

- Consider a drug holiday to reassess the continued effectiveness or necessity of the medication (*see* ADHD, Drug Holidays for details).
- Consider a medication placebo trial if there is an unclear response or if the child, parent, or teacher has strong positive or negative attitudes toward the medication (*see* ADHD, Medication Placebo Trial for details).

Drug Discontinuation:

- Upon withdrawal of the CNS stimulants, the child may experience depressive symptoms or insomnia (Brown, 1985). In addition, rebound or the original symptoms of ADHD may return. There are no published guidelines on tapering the dose of medication. Doses may be tapered over one to two weeks.

SPECIAL INSTRUCTIONS FOR PARENTS/CARE GIVERS/ CHILDREN/ADOLESCENTS

- Stimulant medications are used to help the child/adolescent with schoolwork. Medications need to be used in conjunction with a proper environmental structure, educational assistance, behavioral management, and sometimes individual, family, or group psychotherapy.
- Stimulants should be taken as prescribed. Check with your physician if dosage adjustments are necessary.
- Children may try to take extra medication in order to be a "better child," therefore, medication should be stored in a safe place away from the patient and other children and adolescents. Taking extra doses of the medication can result in overdosage and possible toxicity.
- The extended release dosage forms need to be swallowed whole; do not allow the child to chew the medication, and do not break or crush the medication.
- Administer the medication with or after meals to increase the effectiveness of the medication and to avoid the decrease in appetite.

- If a noontime dose is indicated, encourage discretion on the part of adults who remind the child or administer the dose.
- The most common side effects of the medicine are decreased appetite, stomachaches, insomnia, or headaches. More serious side effects are muscle tics or twitches, or behaviors that are unusual for the child. If this happens, tell the physician right away.
- Do not administer any over-the-counter products without first checking with your physician or pharmacist. Cold and flu products, appetite suppressants, caffeine, or other CNS stimulants should not be taken while on this medicine. Be sure to tell your doctor and pharmacist about any other medications that are being administered.

PRODUCTS AVAILABLE

Standard-Release Dosage Forms

Dextroamphetamine is marketed as Dexedrine® in 5 mg triangular, orange, scored tablets, imprinted with SKF and E19. All of the Dexedrine® products contain tartrazine. Dextroamphetamine is also available in 5 and 10 mg tablets as a generic product

Methylphenidate is marketed as Ritalin® in 5, 10, and 20 mg tablets. Ritalin® 5 mg is a round yellow tablet, imprinted with CIBA 7. Ritalin® 10 mg is a round, pale green scored tablet, imprinted with CIBA 3. Ritalin® 20 mg is a round, pale yellow scored tablet, imprinted with CIBA 34. Generic products are available in the same dosage strengths.

Pemoline, Magnesium is marketed as Cylert® in 18.75, 37.5, and 75 mg scored tablets, and as Cylert Chewable® in 37.5 mg scored tablet. The Cylert® 18.75 mg tablet is white and imprinted with TH. The Cylert® 37.5 mg non-chewable tablet is orange and imprinted with TI. The Cylert® 75 mg tablet is tan and imprinted with TK. The Cylert Chewable® 37.5 mg scored tablet is orange and imprinted with TK.

Extended-Release Dosage Forms

Dextroamphetamine is available as Dexedrine Spansules® in 5, 10, and 15 mg capsules. The 5 mg capsule is imprinted with SKF and E12; the 10 mg capsule is imprinted with SKF and E13; and the 15 mg capsule is imprinted with SKF and E14. The capsules have a brown cap with beige granules. Dexedrine Spansules® also contain tartrazine.

Methylphenidate is available as Ritalin SR® in a 20 mg round, nonscored, white tablet, imprinted with CIBA 16. A generic product is available in the same dosage strength.

COST

GENERIC NAME	TRADENAME	AWP*	AWP* per dose
Dextroamphetamine 5 mg		$19.33 for 100 tablets	$0.19 per tablet
Dextroamphetamine 10 mg		$33.60 for 100 tablets	$0.33 per tablet
Dextroamphetamine	Dexedrine® 5 mg	$18.05 for 100 tablets	$0.18 per tablet
	Dexedrine Spansules® 5 mg	$39.00 for 100 capsules	$0.39 per capsule
	Dexedrine Spansules® 10 mg	$48.70 for 100 capsules	$0.48 per capsule
	Dexedrine Spansules® 15 mg	$62.10 for 100 capsules	$0.62 per capsule
Methylphenidate 5 mg		$25.70 for 100 tablets	$0.25 per tablet
Methylphenidate 10 mg		$35.00 for 100 tablets	$0.35 per tablet
Methylphenidate 20 mg		$50.18 for 100 tablets	$0.50 per tablet
Methylphenidate 20 mg (extended release)		$83.40 for 100 tablets	$0.83 per tablet
Methylphenidate	Ritalin® 5 mg	$29.83 for 100 tablets	$0.29 per tablet
	Ritalin® 10 mg	$42.57 for 100 tablets	$0.42 per tablet
	Ritalin® 20 mg	$61.24 for 100 tablets	$0.61 per tablet
	Ritalin SR® 20 mg	$93.72 for 100 tablets	$0.93 per tablet
Pemoline, Magnesium	Cylert® 18.75 mg	$69.73 for 100 tablets	$0.69 per tablet
	Cylert® 37.5 mg	$109.59 for 100 tablets	$1.09 per tablet
	Cylert® 75 mg	$187.25 for 100 tablets	$1.87 per tablet
	Cylert® 37.5 mg (chewable)	$119.47 for 100 tablets	$1.19 per tablet

* AWP is the average wholesale price to the pharmacist that is listed in the *1994 Redbook* (Cardinale, 1994).

REFERENCES

Abikoff, H, Gittelman, R. The normalizing effects of methylphenidate on the classroom behavior of ADHD children. *J Abnorm Child Psychol,* 1985; 13:33-44.

Ahmann, PA, Waltonen, SJ, Olson, KA, Theye, FW, Van Erem, AJ, LaPlant, RJ. Placebo-controlled evaluation of Ritalin side effects. *Pediatrics,* 1993;91: 1101-1106.

Aman, MG, Marks, RE, Turbott, SH, Wilsher, CP, Merry, SN. Clinical effects of methylphenidate and thioridazine in intellectually subaverage children. *J Am Acad Child Adolesc Psychiatry,* 1991a;30:246-256.

Aman, MG, Marks, RE, Turbott, SH, Wilsher, CP, Merry, SN. Methylphenidate and thioridazine in the treatment of intellectually subaverage children: Effects on cognitive-motor performance. *J Am Acad Child Adolesc Psychiatry,* 1991b;30:816-824.

Barkley, RA. A review of stimulant drug research with hyperactive children. *J Child Psychol Psychiatry,* 1977;18:137-165.

Barkley, RA. The effects of methylphenidate on the interactions of preschool ADHD children with their mothers. *J Am Acad Child Adolesc Psychiatry,* 1988;27:336-341.

Barkley, RA. Hyperactive girls and boys: Stimulant drug effects on mother-child interactions. *J Child Psychol Psych,* 1989b;30:379-390.

Barkley, RA, Karlsson, J, Strzelecki, E, Murphy, JV. Effects of age and ritalin dosage on mother-child interactions of ahyperactive children. *J Consult Clin,* Psychol 1984;52:750-758.

Barkley, RA, McMurray, MB, Edelbrock, CS, Robbins, K. The response of aggressive and nonaggressive ADHD children to two doses of methylphenidate. *J Am Acad Child Adolesc Psychiatry,* 1989a;28:873-881.

Barkley, RA, McMurray, MB, Edelbrock, CS, Robbins, K. Side effects of methylphenidate in children with attention deficit hyperactivity disorder: A systemic, placebo-controlled evaluation. *Pediatrics,* 1990;86:184-192.

Biederman, J, Newcorn, J, Sprich, S. Comorbidity of attention deficit hyperactivity disorder with conduct, depressive, anxiety and other disorders. *Am J Psych,* 1991;148:564-577.

Birmaher, B, Quintana, H, Greenhill, LL. Methylphenidate treatment of hyperactive autistic children. *J Am Acad Child Adolesc Psychiatry,* 1988;27:248-251.

Birmaher, B, Greenhill, LL, Cooper, TB, Fried, J, Maminski, B. Sustained release methylphenidate: Pharmacokinetic studies in ADDH males. *J Am Acad Child Adolesc Psychiatry,* 1989;28:768-772.

Bloom, AS, Russell, LJ, Weisskopf, B, Blackerby, JL. Methylphenidate-induced delusional disorder in a child with attention deficit disorder with hyperactivity. *J Am Acad Child Adolesc Psychiatry,* 1988;27:88-89.

Bradley, C. The behavior of children receiving benzedrine. *Am J Psych,* 1937;94:577-585.

Brown, GL, Ebert, MH, Mikkelsen, EJ, Hunt, RD. Behavior and motor activity response in hyperactive children and plasma amphetamine levels following a sustained release preparation. *J Am Acad Child Psychiatry,* 1980;19:225-239.

Brown, GL, Hunt, RD, Ebert, MH, Bunney, WE, Kopin, IJ. Plasma levels of d-amphetamine in hyperactive children. *Psychopharmacology,* 1979;62:133-140.

Brown, RT. Depression following pemoline withdrawal in a hyperactive child. *Clin Pediatr,* 1985;24:174.

Brown, RT, Sexson, SB. A controlled trial of methylphenidate in black adolescents. *Clin Pediatr,* 1988;27:74-81.

Brown, RT, Sexson, SB. Effects of methylphenidate on cardiovascular responses in attention deficit hyperactivity disordered adolescents. *J Adol Health Care,* 1989;10:179-183.

Brown, RT, Borden, KA, Clingerman, SR. Pharmacotherapy in ADD adolescents with special attention to multimodality treatments. *Psychopharm Bull,* 1985a; 21:192-211.

Brown, RT, Borden, KA, Clingerman, SR. Adherence to methylphenidate therapy in a pediatric population: A preliminary investigation. *Psychopharm Bull,* 1985b;21:28-36.

Cardinale, VA (ed). *1994 Drug Topics Redbook,* Medical Economics Company, Inc., Montvale, NJ, 1994: 154, 163-4, 272, 355.

Chan, YM, Swanson, JM, Soldin, SJ, Thiessen, JJ, MacLeod, SM, Logan, W. Methylphenidate hydrochloride given with or before breakfast: II. Effects on plasma concentration of methylphenidate and ritalinic acid. *Pediatr,* 1983;72:56-59.

Collier, CP, Soldin, SJ, Swanson, JM, MacLeod, SM, Weinberg, F, Rochefort, JG. Pemoline pharmacokinetics and long term therapy in children with attention deficit disorder and hyperactivity. *Clin Pharmacokinetics,* 1985;10:269-278.

Conners, CK. A controlled trial of methylphenidate in preschool children with minimal brain dysfunction. *International J Mental Health,* 1975;4:61-74.

Conners, CK, Barkley, RA. Rating scales and checklists for child psychopharmacology. *Psychopharm Bull,* 1985;21:809-843.

Coons, HW, Klorman, R, Borgstedt, AD. Effects of methylphenidate on adolescents with a childhood history of attention deficit disorder. II. Information processing. *J Am Acad Child Adolesc Psychiatry,* 1987;26:368-374.

Crumrine, PK, Feldman, HM, Toedori, J, Handen, BL, Alvin, RM. The use of methylphenidate in children with seizures and attention deficit disorder. *Ann Neurol,* 1987;22:441-442.

Cunningham, CE, Siegel, LS, Offord, DR. A developmental dose-response analysis of the effects of methylphenidate on the peer interactions of attention deficit disordered boys. *Child Psychol and Psychiatry,* 1985;26:955-971.

Dickinson, LC, Lee, J, Ringdahl, IC, Schedewie, HK, Kilgore, BS, Elders, MJ. Impaired growth in hyperkinetic children receiving pemoline. *J Pediatri,* 1979;94:538-541.

Dulcan, MK. Using psychostimulants to treat behavioral disorders of children and adolescents. *J Child and Adolesc Psychopharmacol,* 1990;1:7-20.

DuPaul, GJ, Rapport, MD. Does methylphenidate normalize the classroom performance of children with attention deficit disorder? *J Am Acad Child Adolesc Psychiatry,* 1993;32:190-198.

Elia, J, Borcherding, BG, Rapoport, JL, Keysor, CS. Methylphenidate and dextroamphetamine treatments of hyperactivity: Are there true nonresponders? *Psych Research,* 1991;36:141-155.

Erenberg, G, Cruse, RP, Rothner, AD. Gilles de la Tourette's syndrome: Effects of stimulant drugs. *Neurology,* 1985;35:1346-1348.

Evans, RW, Gualtieri, CT, Hicks, RE. A neuropathic substrate for stimulant drug effects in hyperactive children. *Clin Neuropharmacol,* 1986;9:264-281.

Evans, SW, Pelham, W. Psychostimulant effects on academic and behavioral measures of ADHD junior high school students in a lecture format classroom. *J Abnormal Child Psychiatry,* 1991;19:537-552.

Famularo, R, Fenton, T. The effect of methylphenidate on school grades in children with attention deficit disorder without hyperactivity: A preliminary report. *J Clin Psych,* 1987;48:112-114.

Feldman, H, Crumrine, P, Handen, BL, Alvin, R, Teodori, J. Methylphenidate in children with seizures and attention-deficit disorder. *AJDC,* 1989;143:1081-1086.

Fine, S, Jewesson, B. Active drug placebo trial of methylphenidate: A clinical service for children with an attention deficit disorder. *Can J Psych,* 1989;34:447-449.

Fine, S, Johnston, C. Drug and placebo side effects in methylphenidate-placebo trial for attention deficit hyperactivity disorder. *Child Psych and Human Dev,* 1993;24:25-30.

Fitzpatrick, PA, Klorman, R, Brumaghim, JT, Borgstedt, AD. Effects of sustained-release and standard preparations of methylphenidate on attention deficit disorder. *J Am Acad Child Adolesc Psychiatry,* 1992;31:226-234.

Friedman, N, Thomas, J, Carr, R, Elders, J, Ringdahl, I, Roche, A. Effect of growth in pemoline-treated children with attention deficit disorder. *Am J Dis Child,* 1981;135:329-332.

Gadow, KD. Effects of stimulant drugs on academic performance in hyperactive and learning disabled children. *J Learning Disabilities,* 1983;16:290-299.

Gadow, KD. Pediatric Psychopharmacology: A review of recent research. *J Child Psychol Psychiatry,* 1992a;33:153-195.

Gadow, KD, Sverd, J. Stimulants for ADHD in child patients with Tourette's syndrome: The issue of relative risk. *J Dev Behav Pediatr,* 1990b;11:269-271.

Gadow, KD, Pomeroy, JC, Nolan, EE. A procedure for monitoring stimulant medication in hyperactive mentally retarded school children. *J Child and Adolecs Psychopharmacology,* 1992c;2:131-143.

Gadow, KD, Nolan, EE, Sverd, J. Methylphenidate in hyperactive boys with comorbid tic disorder: II. Short-term behavioral effects in school settings. *J Am Acad Child Adolesc Psychiatry,* 1992d;31:462-471.

Gadow, KD, Nolan, EE, Sverd, J, Sprafkin, J, Paolicelli, L. Methylphenidate in aggressive-hyperactive boys: I. Effects on peer aggression in public school settings. *J Am Acad Child Adolesc Psychiatry,* 1990a;29:710-718.

Gadow, KD, Paolicelli, LM, Nolan, EE, Schwartz, J, Sprafkin, J, Sverd, J. Methylphenidate in aggressive hyperactive boys: II. Indirect effects of medication treatment on peer behavior. *J Child and Adolecs Psychopharmacology,* 1992b;2:49-60.

Gay, CT, Ryan, SG. Paroxysmal kinesigenic dystonia after methylphenidate administration. *J Child Neurol,* 1994;9:45-46.

Golden, GS. The relationship between stimulant medication and tics. *Pediatr Ann,* 1988;17:405-408.

Greenhill, LL. Pharmacologic treatment of attention deficit hyperactivity disorder. *Psych Clinic North America,* 1992;15:1-27.

Greenhill, LL, Setterberg, S. Pharmacotherapy of disorders of adolescents. *Psych Clinic North Amer,* 1993;16:793-814.

Greenhill, LL, Puig-Antich, J, Novacenko, H. Prolactin, growth hormone and growth responses in boys with attention deficit disorder and hyperactivity treated with methylphenidate. *J Am Acad Child Psychiatry,* 1984;23:58-67.

Greenhill, LL, Cooper, T, Solomon, M, Fried, J, Cornblatt, B. Methylphenidate salivary levels in children. *Psychopharmacol Bull,* 1987;23:115-119.

Grob, CS, Coyle, JT. Suspected adverse methylphenidate-imipramine interactions in children. *Dev Behav Pediatr,* 1986;7:265-267.

Gross, MD. Growth of hyperkinetic children taking methylphenidate, dextroamphetamine or imipramine/desipramine. *Pediatrics,* 1976;58:423-431.

Gualtieri, CT, Hicks, RE. Stimulants and neuroleptics in hyperactive children. *J Amer Acad Child Psych,* 1985;24:363-364.

Gualtieri, CT, Wargin, W, Kanoy, R, Patrick, K, Shen, CD, Youngblood, W, Mueller, RA, Breese, GR. Clinical studies of methylphenidate serum levels in children and adults. *J Am Acad Child Psychiatry,* 1982;21:19-26.

Hagerman, RJ, Murphy, MA, Wittenberger, MD. A controlled trial of stimulant medication in children with the Fragile X syndrome. *Amer J Med Genetics,* 1988;30:377-392.

Halperin, JM, Matier, K, Sarma, V, Newcorn, JH. Specificity of inattention, impulsivitiy and hyperactivity to the diagnosis of attention-deficit hyperactivity disorder. *J Am Acad Child Adolesc Psychiatry,* 1992;31:190-196.

Handen, BL, Feldman, H, Gosling, A, Breaux, AM, McAuliffe, S. Adverse side effects of methylphenidate among mentally retarded children with ADHD. *J Am Acad Child Adolesc Psychiatry,* 1991;30:241-245.

Handen, BL, Breaux, AM, Janosky, J, McAuliffe, S, Feldman, H, Gosling, A. Effects and noneffect of methylphenidate in children with mental retardation and ADHD. *J Am Acad Child Adolesc Psychiatry,* 1992;31:455-461.

Hechtman, L. Adolescent outcome of hyperactive children treated with stimulants in childhood: A review. *Psychopharm Bull,* 1985;21:178-191.

Hinshaw, SP. Stimulant medication and the treatment of aggression in children with attentional deficits. *J Clin Child Psychol,* 1991;20:301-312.

Horn, WF, Ialongo, NS, Pascoe, JM, Greenberg, G, Packard, T, Lopez, M,

Wagner, A, Puttler, L. Additive effects of behavioral parent training, child self-control therapy and stimulant medication with ADHD children. *J Am Acad Child Adolesc Psychiatry*, 1991;30:233-240.

Ialongo, NS, Horn, WF, Pascoe, JM. The effects of multimodal intervention with attention-deficit hyperactivity disorder children: A 9-month follow-up. *J Am Acad Child Adolesc Psychiatry*, 1993;32:182-189.

Jacobvitz, D, Sroufe, LA, Stewart, M, Leffert, N. Treatment of attentional and hyperactivity problems in children with sympathomimetic drugs: A comprehensive review. *J Am Acad Child Adolesc Psychiatry*, 1990;29:677-688.

Johnston, C, Pelham, WE, Hoza, J, Sturges, J. Psychostimulant rebound in attention deficit disordered boys. *J Am Acad Child Adolesc Psychiatry*, 1988;27:806-810.

Kaplan, SL, Busner, J, Kupietz, S, Wasserman, E, Segal, B. Effects of methylphenidate on adolescents with aggressive conduct disorder and ADDH: A preliminary report. *J Am Acad Child Adolesc Psychiatry*, 1990;29:719-724.

Klein, RG, Mannuzza, S. Hyperactive boys almost grown up: III. Methylphenidate effects on ultimate height. *Arch Gen Psych*, 1988b;45:1131-1134.

Klein, RG, Mannuzza, S. Long-term outcome of hyperactive children: A review. *J Am Acad Child Adolesc Psychiatry*, 1991;30:383-387.

Klein, RG, Landa, B, Mattes, JA, Klein, DF. Methylphenidate and growth in hyperactive children: A controlled withdrawal study. *Arch Gen Psych*, 1988a;45:1127-1130.

Klorman, R, Coons, HW, Borgstedt, AD. Effects of methylphenidate on adolescents with a childhood history of attention deficit disorder: I. Clinical findings. *J Am Acad Child Adolesc Psychiatry*, 1987;26:363-367.

Klorman, R, Brumaghim, JT, Fitzpatrick, PA, Borgstedt, AD. Clinical effects of a controlled trial of methylphenidate on adolescents with attention deficit disorder. *J Am Acad Child Adolesc Psychiatry*, 1990;29:702-709.

Koehler-Troy, C, Strober, M, Malenbaum, R. Methylphenidate induced mania in a pre-pubertal child. *J Clin Psych*, 1986;47:566-567.

Licamele, WL. Methylphenidate side effects. *J Am Acad Child Adolesc Psychiatry*, 1988;27:515-516.

Livingston, RL, Dykman, RA, Ackerman, PT. Psychiatric comorbidity and response to two doses of methylphenidate in children with attention deficit disorder. *J Child Adolesc Psychopharmacology*, 1992;2:115-122.

Lou, HC, Henriksen, L, Bruhn, P, Borner, H, Nielsen, JB. Striatal dysfunction in attention deficit and hyperkinetic disorder. *Arch Neurol*, 1989;46:48-52.

Lowe, TL, Cohen, DJ, Detlor, J, Kremenitzer, MW, Shaywitz, BA. Stimulant medications precipitate Tourette's syndrome. *JAMA*, 1982;247:1729-1731.

Lucas, AR, Weiss, M. Methylphenidate hallucinosis. *JAMA*, 1971;217:1079-1081.

Mannuzza, S, Klein, RG, Bessler, A, Malloy, P, LaPadula, M. Adult outcome of hyperactive boys: Educational achievement, occupational rank and psychiatric status. *Arch Gen Psychiatry*, 1993;50:565-576.

Mattes, JA, Gittleman, R. Growth of hyperactive children on maintenance regimen of methylphenidate. *Arch Gen Psych*, 1983;40:317-321.

McBride, MC. An individual double-blind crossover trial for assessing methylphenidate response in children with attention deficit disorder. *J Pediatr,* 1988; 113:137-145.

McBride, MC, Wang, DD, Torres, CF. Methylphenidate in therapeutic doses does not lower seizure threshold. *Ann Neurol,* 1986;20:428.

Patterson, JF. Hepatitis associated with pemoline. *South Med J,* 1984;7:938.

Payton, JB, Burkhart, JE, Hersen, M, Helsel, WJ. Treatment of ADDH in mentally retarded children: A preliminary study. *J Am Acad Child Adolesc Psychiatry,* 1989;28:761-767.

Pelham, WE, Walker, JL, Sturges, J, Hoza, J. Comparative effects of methylphenidate on ADD girls and ADD boys. *J Am Acad Child Adolesc Psychiatry,* 1989; 28:773-776.

Pelham, WE, Bender, ME, Caddell, J, Booth, S, Moorer, SH. Methylphenidate and children with attention deficit disorder: Dose effects on classroom academic and social behavior. *Arch Gen Psych,* 1985;42:948-952.

Pelham, WE, Sturges, J, Hoza, J, Schmidt, C, Bjilsma, JJ, Moorer S. Sustained release and standard methylphenidate effects on cognitive and social behavior in children with attention deficit disorder. *Pediatrics,* 1987;80:491-501.

Pelham, WE, Carlson, C, Sams, SE, Vallano, G, Dixon, MJ, Hoza, B. Separate and combined effects of methylphenidate and behavior modification on boys with attention deficit-hyperactivity disorder in the classroom. *J Consult Clin Psychol,* 1993;61:506-515.

Pelham, WE, Greenslade, KE, Vodde-Hamilton, M, Murphy, DA, Greenstein, JJ, Gnagy, EM, Guthrie, KJ, Hoover, MD, Dahl, RE. Relative efficacy of long-acting stimulants on children with ADHD: A comparison of standard methylphenidate, sustained-release methylphenidate, sustained-release dextroamphetamine, and pemoline. *Pediatrics,* 1990;86:226-237.

Physician's Desk Reference. Oradell, NJ. Medical Economic Data, 1994.

Pliszka, SR. Effect of anxiety on cognition, behavior and stimulant response in ADHD. *J Am Acad Child Adolesc Psychiatry,* 1989;28:882-887.

Pratt, DS, Dubois, RS. Hepatotoxicity due to pemoline: A report of two cases. *J Pediatr Gastroenterol Nutr,* 1990;10:239-241.

Rapoport, JL, Buchsbaum, MS, Weingartner, H, Zahn, TP, Ludlow, C, Mikkelsen, EJ. Dextroamphetamine: Its cognitive and behavioral effects in normal and hyperactive boys and normal men. *Arch Gen Psychiatry,* 1980; 37:933-943.

Rapport, MD, DuPaul, GJ, Kelly, KL. Attention deficit hyperactivity disorder and methylphenidate: The relationship between gross body weight and drug response in children. *Psychopharmacology Bull,* 1989;25:285-290.

Rapport, MD, Quinn, SO, DuPaul, GJ, Quinn, EP, Kelly, KL. Attention deficit disorder with hyperactivity and methylphenidate: The effects of dose and mastery level on children's learning performance. *J Abnormal Child Psych,* 1989;17:669-689.

Rosse, RB, Licamele, WL. Slow-release methylphenidate: Problems when children chew tablets. *J Clin Psych,* 1984;45:525.

Rubenstein, S, Silver, LB, Licamele, WL. Clonidine for stimulant-related sleep problems. *J Am Acad Child Adolesc Psychiatry,* 1994;33:281-282.

Safer, DJ. Relative cardiovascular safety of psychostimulants used to treat attention-deficit hyperactivity disorder. *J Child Adolesc Psychopharmacology,* 1992;2:279-290.

Safer, DJ, Allen, RP. Absence of tolerance to the behavioral effects of methylphenidate in hyperactive and inattentive children. *J Pediatr,* 1989;115:1003-1008.

Safer, DJ, Allen, RP, Barr, E. Depression of growth in hyperactive children on stimulant drugs. *NEJM,* 1972;287:217-220.

Sallee, F, Stiller, R, Perel, J, Bates, T. Oral pemoline kinetics in hyperactive children. *Clin Pharmacol Ther,* 1985;37:606-609.

Sallee, FR, Stiller, RL, Perel, JM. Pharmacodynamics of pemoline in attention deficit disorder with hyperactivity. *J Am Acad Child Adolesc Psychiatry,* 1992;31:244-251.

Sallee, FR, Stiller, RL, Perel, JM, Everett, G. Pemoline-induced abnormal involuntary movement. *J Clin Psychopharmacol,* 1989;9:125-129.

Satterfield, J, Swanson, J, Schell, A, Lee, F. Prediction of antisocial behavior in attention-deficit hyperactivity disorder boys from aggression/defiance scores. *J Am Acad Child Adolesc Psychiatry,* 1994;33:185-190.

Satterfield, JH, Cantwell, DP, Schell, A, Blaschke, T. Growth of hyperactive children treated with methylphenidate. *Arch Gen Psych,* 1979;36:212-217.

Schachar, R, Tannock, R. Childhood hyperactivity and psychostimulants: A review of extended treatment studies. *J Child and Adolesc Psychopharmacology,* 1993;3:81-97.

Schachar, R, Taylor, E, Wieselberg, M, Thorley, G, Rutter, M. Changes in family function and relationships in children who respond to methylphenidate. *J Am Acad Child Adolesc Psychiatry,* 1987;26:728-729.

Schleifer, M, Weiss, G, Cohen, N, Elman, M, Cvejic, H, Kruger, E. Hyperactivity in preschoolers and the effect of methylphenidate. *Am J Orthopsychiatry,* 1975;45:38-50.

Shaywitz, BA, Shaywitz, SE, Sebrechts, MM, Anderson, GM, Cohen, DJ, Jatlow, P, Young, JG. Growth hormone and prolactin response to methylphenidate in children with attention deficit disorder. *Life Sci,* 1990;46:625-633.

Shaywitz, SE, Hunt, RD, Jatlow, P. Psychopharmacology of attention deficit disorder: Pharmacokinetic, neuroendocrine and behavioral measures following acute and chronic treatment with methylphenidate. *Pediatrics,* 1982;69:688-694.

Speltz, ML, Varley, CK, Peterson, K, Beilke, RL. Effects of dextroamphetamine and contingency management on a preschooler with ADHD and oppositional defiant disorder. *J Am Acad Child Adolesc Psychiatry,* 1988;27:175-178.

Sprague, RL, Sleator, EK. Methylphenidate in hyperkinetic children: Differences in dose effects on learning and social behavior. *Science,* 1977;198:1274-1276.

Strayhorn, JM, Rapp, N, Donina, W, Strain, PS. Randomized trial of methylphenidate for an autistic child. *J Am Acad Child Adolesc Psychiatry,* 1988;27: 244-247.

Swanson, JM, Sandman, CA, Deutsch, C, Baien, M. Methylphenidate hydrochloride given with or before breakfast. I. Behavioral, cognitive, and electrophysiologic effects. *Pediatrics,* 1983;72:49-55.

Tannock, R, Schachar, R. Methylphenidate and cognitive perseveration in hyperactive children. *J Child Psychol Psych,* 1992;33:1217-1228.

United States Pharmacopeia, Drug Information, 1994, Volumes I and II. Sections on methylphenidate, amphetamines, and pemoline.

Varley, CK. Effects of methylphenidate in adolescents with attention deficit disorder. *J Am Acad Child Psychiatry,* 1983;22:351-354.

Varley, CK. A review of studies of drug treatment efficacy for attention deficit disorder with hyperactivity in adolescents. *Psychopharm Bull,* 1985; 21:216-221.

Vincent, J, Varley, CK, Leger, P. Effects of methylphenidate on early adolescent growth. *Am J Psych,* 1990;147:501-502.

Whalen, CK, Henker, B, Buhrmester, D, Hinshaw, SP, Huber, A, Laski, K. Does stimulant medication improve the peer status of hyperactive children? *J Consult Clin Psychol,* 1989;57:545-549.

Wilens, TE, Biederman, J. The Stimulants. *Psych Clinic North Amer,* 1992;14:191-222.

Zametkin, AJ, Rapoport JL. Neurobiology of attention deficit disorder with hyperactivity: Where have we come in 50 years? *J Am Acad Child Adolesc Psychiatry,* 1987;26:676-686.

Zametkin, AJ, Borcherding, BG. The neuropharmacology of attention-deficit hyperactivity disorder. *Ann Rev Med,* 1989;40:447-451.

Chapter 2

Antidepressants

TRICYCLIC ANTIDEPRESSANTS

Amitriptyline hydrochloride

    Elavil® is marketed by Stuart Pharmaceuticals.

    Endep® is marketed by Roche Laboratories.

    Amitriptyline is also available in generic form.

Clomipramine hydrochloride

    Anafranil® is marketed by Ciba Geigy Pharmaceuticals.

Desipramine hydrochloride

    Norpramin® is marketed by Marion Merrell Dow.

    Desipramine is also available in generic form.

Imipramine hydrochloride

    Janimine® is marketed by Abbott Laboratories.

    Tofranil® is marketed by Ciba Geigy Pharmaceuticals.

    Imipramine is also available in generic form.

Nortriptyline hydrochloride

    Aventyl® is marketed by Eli Lilly

    Pamelor® is marketed by Sandoz Pharmaceuticals.

    Nortriptyline is also available in generic form.

DSM-IV INDICATIONS

Enuresis

Attention-Deficit/Hyperactivity Disorder (??)*

Depression (???)**

Separation Anxiety Disorder (???)

Obsessive Compulsive Disorder (??)

> FDA: Amitriptyline, desipramine, and nortriptyline are approved for depression in adolescents. Imipramine hydrochloride (not the pamoate formulation) is approved for children six years of age and older for enuresis and for adolescents in the treatment of depression. Clomipramine is approved for use in children older than ten years in the treatment of obsessive compulsive disorder (*PDR*, 1994).

> USP: The effectiveness of the tricyclic antidepressants has not been established in the treatment of depression in children and adolescents; amitriptyline, desipramine, imipramine and nortriptyline have been used. Imipramine hydrochloride (not the pamoate) and amitriptyline are indicated in the treatment of nocturnal enuresis in children over the age of six years. Imipramine and desipramine are being used in the treatment of attention-deficit/ hyperactivity disorder (ADHD) in children over six years of age; however, deaths have been reported in children treated with desipramine for ADHD (*USPDI,* 1994).

* Two question marks (??) signify preliminary information is limited but that a positive effect has been suggested by one or more investigators.

** Three question marks (???) signify that the information is very preliminary and efficacy is questionable, or a lack of efficacy has been reported.

Refer to the Preface for a full explanation of the question marks.

CONTRAINDICATIONS: Hypersensitivity to tricyclic antidepressants; hypersensitivity to agents with a tricyclic chemical structure, such as carbamazepine; bipolar disorder (*see* Adverse Effects,

Rapid cycling); cardiovascular disorders; hepatic/renal function impairment; hyperthyroidism; psychosis, schizophrenia; hypersensitivity to tartrazine (Janimine®); asthma (Kanner et al., 1989).

PHARMACOLOGY: Tricyclic antidepressants increase the synaptic concentrations of norepinephrine and serotonin in the central nervous system by inhibiting the reuptake of the neurotransmitters into the presynaptic neuron. Amitriptyline and clomipramine are more potent inhibitors of the reuptake of serotonin, however, their secondary metabolites are inhibitors of the reuptake of norepinephrine. Desipramine and nortriptyline are inhibitors of the reuptake of norepinephrine. Imipramine inhibits both serotonin and norepinephrine reuptake. The tricyclic antidepressants are associated with high anticholinergic effects in the periphery and central nervous system and have sedative, antihistaminic, and antiarrhythmic effects.

STUDIES OF TRICYCLIC ANTIDEPRESSANT EFFICACY

Enuresis

Enuresis is the involuntary discharge of urine after bladder control is expected to have been attained. Nocturnal enuresis, or bedwetting, is present in 10 to 15 percent of five year olds, 7 percent of ten year olds, and 1 percent of adults. There is a spontaneous cure rate of 15 percent per year after the age of six (Forsythe and Redmond, 1974). The treatment of choice is the enuresis alarm, which is the only therapy proven to provide a lasting cure. Random awakenings to empty the bladder are not effective in the treatment of nocturnal enuresis (Fournier et al., 1987). Drug therapy is indicated when an adequate trial of bladder training or the bed-wetting alarm methods fail. Exceptions to this general guideline are when the parents or caretakers are very impatient with the slow process of nondrug methods or the child is at risk of physical or psychological harm.

Tricyclic antidepressants (TCA-D) are effective in reducing the frequency of enuretic episodes, however, total remission is infrequent (10 to 20 percent of patients), and discontinuation of the drug frequently leads to relapse. The mechanism of action in the treatment of enuresis is unknown but may be related to the anticholinergic effect that increases functional bladder capacity or possibly to an increase in antidiuretic hormone. The mechanism of action is probably not related to an antidepressant effect (Miller, Atkin, and Moody, 1992). For children six years of age and older, imipramine is approved by the Food and Drug Administration for the treatment of enuresis, but desipramine, amitriptyline, and nortriptyline are also effective. Patients are usually treated for three to six months and then the medication is gradually discontinued to avoid relapse.

For children six years and older, the initial dose of imipramine should be 25 mg at bedtime, with weekly increases of 25 mg per night, if necessary. One week is needed to evaluate the efficacy of a new dose. A nightly dose greater than 75 mg is rarely necessary for children, however, doses up to 175 mg have been required in teenagers (Fritz, Rockney, and Yeung, 1994). The anti-enuretic effect is often immediate and is usually evident within seven days. An initially effective dose often becomes ineffective in two to six weeks, but increasing the dose usually reestablishes control. Efficacy ratings vary, but total elimination of bed-wetting is infrequent. Fritz, Rockney, and Yeung (1994) reported that four of 18 patients became totally dry while taking imipramine 2.5 mg/kg per night. Ten of 18 were partial responders with 62 to 82 percent with dry nights, and four of 18 patients were nonresponders.

This study suggests that imipramine and desipramine plasma concentrations correlate with clinical response, a finding that has been reported (Fernandez de Gatta et al., 1990; Furlanut et al., 1989; Rapoport et al., 1980) and disputed (Fournier et al., 1987) previously. At doses of imipramine 1.0 mg/kg, the group of children had 54.8 percent dry nights. With increases in 0.5 mg/kg per night, the percentage of dry nights was 62.4 percent, 64.8 percent, and 73 percent, respectively (Fritz, Rockney, and Yeung, 1994). There was a 700 percent variation between the highest and lowest blood level at each weight determined equivalent dose. Higher doses or plasma levels are not associated with an increased rate of complete dryness. The authors suggest that plasma levels may have a role in determining low blood levels, toxicity, or noncompliance.

Depression

Currently, none of the double-blind placebo-controlled studies of the use of tricyclic antidepressants (TCA-D) in the treatment of depression in children (Geller et al., 1989; Kashani, Shekim, and Reid, 1984; Petti and Law, 1982; Puig-Antich et al., 1987) or adolescents (Boulos et al., 1991; Geller et al., 1990; Kramer and Feiguine, 1981; Kutcher et al., 1994) have found medication to be superior to placebo. There are numerous proposed reasons for these findings. First, the TCA-D have been studied in very few children or adolescents, suggesting that with further research, a positive effect may be observed. Second, the diagnostic criteria and rating scales used for adult depression may not reflect depression or response in the pediatric population. Third, children and adolescents with major depression may represent a heterogeneous sample with physiological differences. Fourth, children and adolescents may have differences in neurotransmission, possibly due to differences in sex hormone levels, resulting in a nonresponse. Fifth, major depression in the younger population may be a more severe illness, nonresponsive to current therapies.

Overall, practitioners and researchers consider the efficacy of the tricyclic antidepressants to be an open question (Ambrosini et al., 1993; Gadow, 1992; Jensen, Ryan, and Prien, 1992; Strober, 1992). Tricyclic antidepressants should be used in the treatment of child and adolescent depression only after careful consideration of the lack of superiority over placebo and the risk of adverse effects.

Attention-Deficit/Hyperactivity Disorder

The central nervous system (CNS) stimulants are the drugs of choice in the treatment of attention-deficit/hyperactivity disorder (ADHD). The tricyclic antidepressants are alternative agents in the treatment of ADHD. The TCA-D are indicated when the patient does not respond to the CNS stimulants or has concurrent symptoms of ADHD and anxiety, depression, enuresis, or sleep disturbances (Pliszka, 1987), although patients without comorbidity also respond to TCA-D therapy (Biederman et al., 1993a). The use of a tricyclic antidepressant has several potential benefits including a longer duration of action into the evening hours (beneficial for parents), less sleep disturbance, and reduced risk of abuse (Biederman, 1988). The negative aspects of using the TCA-D for ADHD include increased risk of toxicity with overdose, negative cognitive effects, increased side effects, and increased noncompliance. Of the four cases of sudden death associated with desipramine therapy, three of the cases were taking desipramine for ADHD (*see* Adverse Reactions/Case Reports).

In comparison studies of TCA-D and stimulants, the stimulants are rated superior, but low doses of the TCA-D have been used. In the study, by Rapoport et al. (1974), a mean dose of imipramine 80 mg per day was compared to methylphenidate 20 mg per day. Garfinkel et al. (1983) used a mean dose of 85 mg per day of clomipramine or desipramine in comparison to a mean dose of 18 mg per day of methylphenidate. Higher doses of the TCA-D may have been more effective, although a one year follow-up study of the Rapoport et al. (1974) study indicates a higher rate of discontinuance with low dose imipramine therapy (Quinn and Rapoport, 1975). Open studies indicate that imipramine (Cox, 1982), desipramine (Biederman, Gastfriend, and Jellinek, 1986; Gastfriend, Biederman, and Jellinek, 1984), and nortriptyline (Saul, 1985) are effective in the treatment of ADHD.

In the report by Saul (1985), 54 out of 60 children were treated with nortriptyline up to 75 mg per day. Each of the children were nonresponders or developed adverse effects to the CNS stimulants, or had concurrent symptoms of depression. Nortriptyline therapy was associated with a change in attitude, followed by an increase in attention span and a decrease in impulsivity. In a retrospective chart review conducted by Wilens et al. (1993a), nortriptyline was effective in 76 percent of 58 treatment resistant cases of ADHD. Thirty-seven children (ages seven to 12 years old) and 21 adolescents (ages 13 to 18 years old) were included. Eighty-four percent of the patients had at least one comorbid diagnosis. Nortriptyline doses ranged from 20 to 200 mg per day (mean of 73.6 mg per day), or 0.4 to 4.5 mg/kg/day (mean of 1.94 mg/kg/day). Adverse effects associated with nortriptyline include lethargy, gastrointestinal distress, weight gain, symptomatic orthostatic hypotension, insomnia, and increased agitation. The therapeutic response to nortriptyline was observed within two to four weeks of treatment and was sustained for a mean of 15 months. Further prospective-controlled studies are needed to evaluate the role of nortriptyline in the treatment of ADHD.

Rapoport et al. (1985) reported a two week double-blind, placebo-controlled study of desipramine in 29 boys, ages six to 12 years old (mean age of 8.8 years). The mean desipramine doses used were 98.7 mg per day or 3.4 mg/kg/day. Clinical effects were observed within three days of desipramine therapy. The positive effects observed at the end of the trial did not correlate with plasma concentrations of desipramine or the hydroxy-desipramine metabolite. In addition, Donnelly et al. (1986) reported a two week, double-blind, placebo-controlled trial of 29 boys (mean age of 8.8 years) with ADHD. After a one-week baseline period, the patients were randomly assigned to a single daily dose of desipramine 25 to 100 mg per day (mean of 3.38 mg/kg/day) or placebo. Desipramine therapy resulted in an immediate improvement in classroom motor activity, however, there were no changes in cognitive tasks. Desipramine therapy was associated with a ten beats per minute increase in heart rate and a 10 mm Hg increase in both supine systolic and standing diastolic blood pressure. There was a six to ten fold variation in plasma concentrations of desipramine and its metabolites that did not correlate with response, dose, or changes in blood pressure or pulse. In this study, the plasma levels were drawn 20 to 24 hours after the single daily dose and probably are not accurate measurements considering the shorter half-life of desipramine in children.

Biederman et al. (1989a) reported on the use of desipramine in 42 children (less than 12 years of age) and 20 adolescents (12 years and older) who responded poorly to central nervous system stimulants. Patients with mental retardation (full scale IQ < 70), psychosis, autism, or other medical or neurological disorders were excluded from the study. During the six-week double-blind, placebo-controlled study, no other psychotropics or formal psychological or behavioral therapy was administered. At the end of three to six weeks of the study, 68 percent of the desipramine patients were much to very much improved on the Clinical Global Improvement scale compared to only 10 percent of the patients on placebo. Three to four weeks of therapy were required to reach a significant desipramine (mean dose of 4.6 mg/kg/day) versus placebo difference in benefits.

There was no significant difference on cognitive measures between desipramine and placebo.

The adverse effects reported are dry mouth, decreased appetite, headaches, abdominal discomfort, tiredness, dizziness, trouble sleeping, and weight loss. Serum desipramine levels varied an average of 16.5 fold and ranged from 22 to 896 ng/ml, with a mean serum level of 227 ng/ml. There was no significant linear relationship between serum desipramine levels and total or weight adjusted daily doses. In addition, no clinically significant linear association was found between serum levels and therapeutic response. Desipramine therapy was associated with clinically asymptomatic but statistically significant increases in diastolic blood pressure, heart rate, and intraventricular conduction defect of the right bundle branch block type (RBBB). Two patients developed complete RBBB. The authors indicate that TCA-D therapy for children with ADHD can be effective and safe, but requires careful monitoring of the TCA-D serum levels and cardiovascular functioning.

Uncontrolled studies of patients with concurrent ADHD and Tourette's syndrome have reported a marked reduction in the symptoms of ADHD with desipramine (Riddle et al., 1988; Spencer et al., 1993a) or nortriptyline (Spencer et al., 1993b) therapy. In these uncontrolled case reports, there was no exacerbation in tics, however, the development of tics with imipramine therapy has been reported (Parraga and Cochran, 1992). Further studies are needed to determine the role of the tricyclic antidepressants in the treatment of ADHD with or without comorbid disorder. Subsequent studies should compare central nervous system stimulants to the tricyclic antidepressants at the higher doses currently used in the treatment of ADHD. In consideration of the case reports of sudden death with desipramine, future research studies will require tightly controlled methodology to determine the efficacy and adverse effects in this population of patients. Judicious use of the TCA-D in the treatment of ADHD is indicated until the safety of these agents is fully investigated (*see* Adverse Reactions/Case Reports).

Separation Anxiety Disorder/School Phobia

Although there is limited information on the use of the tricyclic antidepressants (TCA-D) in the treatment of separation anxiety, or school phobia, controlled studies suggest that the TCA-D are no more effective than placebo. Klein and Klein (1971) reported a six-week, double-blind, placebo-controlled study of 35 outpatients aged six to 14 years (mean age of 10.8 years) treated with imipramine 100 to 200 mg per day (mean of 152 mg/day). Both treatment groups received psychotherapy. There was a high improvement rate with placebo but imipramine was statistically superior on several ratings scales. The only adverse effect that occurred more frequently in the imipramine treated group was dry mouth. A subsequent six-week study (Klein, Koplewicz, and Kanner, 1992) failed to show a significant difference between imipramine and placebo in 20 children, aged six to 15 years (mean age of 9.5 years). Imipramine was titrated to a maximum of 5 mg/kg/day and resulted in doses ranging from 75 to 275 mg per day (mean of 153 mg per day). Children received weekly behavioral treatment during the study. Frequent adverse effects associated with imipramine were irritability and angry outbursts.

Berney et al. (1981) conducted a 12-week, double-blind, placebo-controlled trial in 46 subjects; 28 were adolescents (over 12 years of age), and 18 were pre-adolescent (younger than 12 years old). The dose of clomipramine was 40 mg for nine and ten year olds, 50 mg for 11 and 12 year olds, and 75 mg for 13 and 14 year olds per day. Clomipramine and placebo were found equally ineffective in reducing the symptoms of separation anxiety. Higher doses of clomipramine will potentially result in more positive results.

Bernstein, Garfinkel, and Borchardt (1990) conducted a double-blind, placebo-controlled comparison of alprazolam to imipramine in 24 children or adolescents, aged 7.66 to 17.58 years (mean of 14.12 years). Patients with diagnoses of major depression, adjustment disorder with depressed mood, separation anxiety disorder and/or overanxious disorder, or a combination of these disorders were included. Patients were randomly assigned to 0.03 mg/kg/day of alprazolam, 3 mg/kg/day of imipramine, or placebo. Medication was administered in three divided daily doses. Results showed no significant difference between the three groups. Adverse effects associated with drug therapy were blurred vision, constipation, dry mouth, dizziness, and dizziness upon standing. Further research of patients with separation anxiety disorder is needed to determine the role of medication therapy in this treatment-resistant disorder (*see also* Attention-Deficit/Hyperactivity Disorder for further information on anxiety disorders and response to tricyclic antidepressants).

Obsessive Compulsive Disorder

Flament et al. (1985) reported a double-blind, placebo-controlled crossover trial of clomipramine in 19 patients with severe treatment-resistant obsessive compulsive disorder (OCD). The patients were ten to 18 years old (mean of 14.5 years) and did not have symptoms of psychosis, neurological abnormalities, or mental retardation. Patients were excluded from the study if they had a primary affective disorder but were included if the patient had depression secondary to OCD. The duration of OCD prior to the study ranged from one to ten years with an average of four years. Patients were randomly assigned to placebo or clomipramine for five weeks before crossing over to the other group.

Patients were started at clomipramine 50 mg and increased by 50 per day up to a maximum of 3 mg/kg/day or 200 mg/day. Patients received individual supportive psychotherapy, but no behavioral therapy. At the completion of the five weeks, the average dose of clomipramine was 141 mg per day (range of 100 to 200 mg per day). Plasma levels of clomipramine did not correlate with measures of symptom change. Patient improvement was rated by the reduction in symptoms. Of the 19 patients, 42 percent showed a 50 percent or more reduction in symptoms, and 74 percent showed at least a 25 percent or more reduction in symptoms. Patients with rituals tended to respond better than patients with the obsessional type of OCD. Two patients had a virtually total resolution in symptoms. Adverse effects were tremor, dry mouth, dizziness, constipation, acute dyskinesia, tonic-clonic seizure (one patient), psychotic reaction, heart pounding, blurred vision, increased salivation, and difficulty urinating.

Leonard et al. (1989) conducted a double-blind, crossover study of clomipramine and desipramine in 48 patients (age range of seven to 19 years, mean of 13.9 years) with severe OCD. The outpatient trial began with a two-week single-blind, placebo phase followed by randomization to begin either clomipramine or desipramine. Desipramine was selected as the comparison drug to clomipramine to compare a selective noradrenergic tricyclic antidepressant with clomipramine, a tricyclic antidepressant selective for serotonin. The initial dose of either drug during the five-week treatment period was either 25 or 50 mg increased to a maximum of 5 mg/kg/day or 250 mg/day.

The physician ratings indicated that clomipramine is superior to desipramine in ameliorating symptoms of OCD at five weeks of treatment; however, there was no difference in the child self-ratings for desipramine versus clomipramine. The final mean dose of clomipramine was 150 mg/day (3.0 mg/kg/day) and 153 mg/day (3.0 mg/kg/day) for desipramine. Adverse effects included dry mouth, tremor, constipation, difficulty urinating, dizziness, and sweating. Clomipramine was also associated with chest pain, hot flashes, heartburn, rash, and acne. Two patients were discontinued from the trial due to the development of psychosis and depression, one each for clomipramine and desipramine. A subsequent report described the double-blind substitution of desipramine for long-term clomipramine that resulted in the relapse of eight out nine patients (Leonard et al., 1991). The authors acknowledge that the symptoms of OCD vary in severity over time and suggest that long-term therapy may be required in clomipramine responsive patients.

DeVeaugh-Geiss et al. (1992) conducted a multicenter, double-blind, placebo-controlled study of clomipramine in 60 patients, ten to 17 years old (mean age of 14.5 years). For the first two weeks all patients received placebo, followed by random assignment to placebo or clomipramine for eight weeks. Clomipramine 25 mg was administered for the first four days and followed by gradual titration to a minimum of 75 mg daily, or maximum of 3 mg/kg/day or 200 mg/day. No other psychotropic drugs were administered with the exception of chloral hydrate. Supportive psychotherapy was allowed but behavioral therapy was excluded. Clomipramine therapy was associated with a 34 percent reduction in symptoms of OCD compared to an 8 percent reduction with placebo. The open label extension of this trial suggests that patients may continue to improve on clomipramine therapy with a further reduction in symptoms of OCD. Adverse effects included palpitation, elevated liver enzymes requiring discontinuation of clomipramine, mild increase in pulse, reductions in systolic blood pressure, dry mouth, somnolence, dizziness, fatigue, tremor, constipation, anorexia, and dyspepsia.

The above studies suggest that clomipramine is superior to placebo in the treatment of OCD, however further studies are needed to determine the efficacy of clomipramine in comparison to behavioral treatment methods. To determine whether the adverse effects of clomipramine are more frequent or more severe than those associated with other tricyclic antidepressants, further assessment is needed.

DEVELOPMENTAL PHARMACOKINETICS

Absorption: In adults, imipramine and amitriptyline are generally rapidly absorbed with peak plasma levels at one to three hours after ingestion. Desipramine and nortriptyline are absorbed more slowly with peak levels at four to eight hours after ingestion (Preskorn, 1993).

Metabolism: Tricyclic antidepressants are extensively metabolized by hepatic oxidation, aromatic hydroxylation, and demethylation. Children may have less hepatic isoenzyme, cytochrome P4502D6, than adults, which suggests that children may have proportionally less secondary metabolites than adults (Wilens et al., 1993b). Cytochrome P4502D6 is the enzyme that converts the tricyclic antidepressants to active and inactive metabolites. Five to 10 percent of the Caucasian population are poor metabolizers of the tricyclic antidepressants and lack the cytochrome P4502D6 enzyme. These "slow hydroxylators" will have much longer half-lives and higher blood levels of the TCA-D. Amitriptyline is metabolized to nortriptyline and other metabolites. Imipramine is metabolized to desipramine and other metabolites.

Half-life: Geller et al. (1984) reported the mean half-life of nortriptyline in prepubertal patients as 17.6 hours with a range of 13.6 to 24.1 hours. The mean half-life of nortriptyline in postpubertal patients was 27.1 hours with a range of 14.2 to 76.2 hours (Geller et al., 1984).

Plasma levels: A fixed dose of a tricyclic antidepressant will result in a six- to 72-fold variation in steady state plasma levels of the tricyclic antidepressant and of the secondary metabolites. The variation is due to interindividual variations in the rate of metabolism (Preskorn et al., 1989; Fetner and Geller, 1992). Preskorn et al. (1989) reported the finding that in 68 children (aged six to 14 years) taking imipramine, 80 percent had desipramine (a secondary metabolite of imipramine) plasma levels that exceeded imipramine levels. This finding suggests that children have a relatively high serum desipramine/imipramine ratio. Several studies have failed to show a relationship between desipramine or nortriptyline plasma levels and antidepressant response (Geller et al., 1992; Kutcher et al., 1994; Olig et al., 1985; Ryan et al., 1986). However, Preskorn, Weller, and Weller (1982) and Puig-Antich et al. (1987) suggest that children have a higher rate of antidepressant response if the total imipramine plus desipramine levels are between 125 to 225 ng/ml. Plasma levels of the tricyclic antidepressants are drawn ten to 12 hours after the last dose, usually in the morning.

DOSAGE RANGES

Due to the lack of correlation between dose and resulting plasma levels, dosing of the TCA-D should be according to patient response, adverse effects, and plasma levels. A TCA-D dose based on the weight of the patient will result in unpredictable plasma levels. The lowest effective dose should be utilized to avoid possible adverse effects. Higher doses of the TCA-D are associated with an increased incidence of cardiac and central nervous system adverse effects. Children and adolescents are usually administered two divided daily doses of the TCA-D, however some adolescents may be able to take a single daily dose.

> **Enuresis:** Imipramine doses greater than 2.5 mg/kg/day are not recommended. For children six years and older, the initial dose of imipramine should be 25 mg at bedtime, with weekly increases of 25 mg per night, if necessary. One week is needed to evaluate the efficacy of a new dose. A nightly dose greater than 75 mg is rarely neces-

sary for children, however, doses up to 175 mg have been required in teenagers (Fritz, Rockney, and Yeung, 1994). The anti-enuretic effect is often immediate and is usually evident within seven days. An initially effective dose often becomes ineffective in two to six weeks, but increasing the dose usually reestablishes control.

Depression: The tricyclic antidepressants have not been shown to be more effective than placebo in the treatment of depression. Amitriptyline, imipramine, and desipramine have been investigated in children and adolescents up to maximum doses of 5 mg/kg/day, however, adolescents may be more sensitive to the effects of the TCA-D and may not require more than 100 mg per day. Nortriptyline doses of 10 to 140 mg per day (adjusted to plasma levels) have been investigated in the treatment of children and adolescents with depression. Ryan et al. (1987) administered imipramine as a single dose at bedtime after patients were stabilized at steady-state on three times daily dosing. The 29 patients (age 10.8 to 18 years old, mean of 14.7 years) were assessed over the next 24 hours with electrocardiograms and plasma levels of imipramine and desipramine. Although the authors suggest that adolescent patients can be safely converted from a three times a day frequency to a single bedtime dose, precaution is needed. A single dose will result in higher peak blood levels of the tricyclic antidepressant, and considering the unexplained deaths associated with the tricyclic antidepressants, divided daily doses are indicated until further studies are conducted (Fetner and Geller, 1992).

Attention-Deficit/Hyperactivity Disorder: Desipramine doses up to 5 mg/kg per day have been investigated (Biederman et al., 1989a). Nortriptyline doses up to 4.5 mg/kg per day (mean of 1.94 mg/kg/day) have been investigated (Wilens et al., 1993a).

Obsessive-Compulsive Disorder: For children over the age of ten years, doses of clomipramine are initiated at 25 mg per day and increased by 25 to 50 mg every four to seven days to a maximum of 3 mg/kg/day or 200 mg per day for children.

ADVERSE EFFECTS REPORTED IN CHILDREN AND ADOLESCENTS

COMMON

Anticholinergic effects: Dry mouth (alleviated by sucking on hard sugarless candy or chewing sugarless gum), constipation (alleviated by increasing water consumption, diet, bulk producing laxatives like psyllium, and stool softeners), blurred vision, tachycardia, and urinary retention.

Rash: An erythematous, maculopapular, and pruretic rash, frequently develops. Tricyclic antidepressant induced rashes may resolve in a few days, and the TCA-D may or may not require discontinuation (Biederman et al., 1988b).

Cardiovascular effects: The doses or plasma levels of a tricyclic antidepressant do not directly correlate with cardiovascular findings, however, higher plasma levels are associated with an increased incidence of cardiovascular effects (Biederman et al., 1989b; Donnelly et al., 1986; Preskorn et al., 1983). Postural hypotension, hypertension, increased intraventricular conduction time, QRS complex widening, PR interval lengthening (delayed cardiac conduction), prolonged QT interval, T-wave flattening, tachycardia, class 1A quinidine-like and class 1B lidocaine-like antiarrhythmic effects may occur (Kuekes et al., 1992; Mosholder, Wooldridge, and Bates, 1989). The most common cardiovascular findings are increased PR interval, increased heart rate, and widening of the QRS complex (Bartels et al., 1991; Biederman et al., 1989b; Fletcher et al., 1993; Schroeder et al., 1989; Wilens et al., 1993c; Winsberg et al., 1975). Right bundle branch block is frequently found in the pediatric population on the baseline electrocardiogram. Patients may complain of heart pounding or chest pain. Patients require baseline and follow-up assessment to monitor the effects of the tricyclic antidepressants on cardiovascular functioning (*see* Adverse Reactions/Case Reports).

Central nervous system: Irritability, headache, tiredness, lethargy, insomnia, and dizziness.

Other adverse effects: Anorexia, weight growth reduction (Spencer et al., 1992), weight gain, and gastrointestinal distress.

LESS COMMON (*see also* Adverse Reactions/Case Reports)

Rapid cycling: Rapid cycling is defined as more than four mood episodes per year. Tricyclic antidepressants may induce rapid cycling in patients with a family history of bipolar disorder (Ghadirian and Kusalic, 1990). Akiskal and Mallya (1987) suggest that patients who are bipolar or have a family history of bipolar disorder are at risk of developing rapid cycling with prolonged use of tricyclic antidepressants.

Central nervous system effects: Confusional states, disorientation, impaired concentration/attention, agitation, rage reactions, social withdrawal (Preskorn et al., 1983; Preskorn et al., 1988), induction of mania (Geller, Fox, and Fletcher, 1993) or psychosis, including delusions or hallucinations (Alarcon, Johnson, and Lucas, 1991; Preskorn et al., 1983; Preskorn, et al. 1988), peripheral neurological symptoms (Stept and Subramony, 1988), tics (Parraga and Cochran, 1992), self-abusive behavior (Cruz, 1992), acute dyskinesia (Flament et al., 1985), tremor and seizures (more frequently found in patients with neurological disorders or abnormal electroencephalograms) have been reported. Higher plasma levels of the TCA-D are associated with an increased incidence of central nervous system adverse effects (Preskorn et al., 1983; Preskorn et al., 1988).

Other adverse effects: Height growth reduction (Spencer et al., 1992), racing thoughts (Gastfriend, Biederman, and Jellinek, 1984), photosensitization, hot flashes, acne, and increased liver function tests.

ALLERGIC REACTION: Patients can develop an allergic cutaneous skin reaction that may or may not require discontinuation of the TCA-D (Biederman, 1988b). In addition, some formulations of the tricyclic antidepressants contain tartrazine (FD&C Yellow No. 5 dye) which can cause an allergic reaction. Tartrazine hypersensitivity is more likely to occur in patients with aspirin hypersensitivity.

TOXICITY: Symptoms include drowsiness, delirium (disorientation, forgetfulness, agitation, insomnia), stupor, coma, rigidity, athetoid and choreiform movements, convulsions, arrhythmias, tachycardia, congestive heart failure, respiratory depression, hypotension, hyperpyrexia, mydriasis, and diaphoresis. The risk of mortality associated with TCA-D overdose is very high.

ADVERSE REACTIONS/CASE REPORTS

Tricyclic Antidepressants Associated with Sudden Death

In 1990, the Medical Letter® reported three cases of sudden death with desipramine therapy (Abramowicz, 1990). A fourth case was subsequently reported by Riddle, Geller, and Ryan (1993). All four cases involved children exposed to desipramine therapy, however, none of the evidence suggests a single, direct etiological factor. Three of the children were treated for attention-deficit/hyperactivity disorder (ADHD), and one child was treated for depression. Two of the children were taking unknown doses of desipramine and two cases were taking either 3.15 mg/kg/day or 2.56 mg/kg/day. One child, after playing tennis, took a nap and was later found unconscious in her bed. One child collapsed after running laps in the gymnasium, and two of the children collapsed at home or at school. The events leading to the collapse of these two children was not specified or reported. Several hypotheses have been proposed to explain these findings. Of the tricyclic depressants, desipramine is the most specific inhibitor of norepinephrine reuptake. This inhibition of reuptake of norepinephrine increases cardiac sympathetic tone, which may predipose the patient to developing ventricular tachyarrhythmias, syncope, and sudden death (Riddle, Geller, and Ryan, 1993). In addition, patients taking desipramine may develop the long QT syndrome found on the electrocardiogram. The long QT syndrome can lead to polymorphic ventricular tachyarrhythmias, referred to as Torsades de pointes (Riddle et al., 1991). Other hypotheses include a direct toxic effect of desipramine or its metabolites on cardiac tissue, preexisting cardiac abnormalities, and the possibility that these sudden deaths were a chance occurrence (Riddle et al., 1991).

Biederman et al. (1993b) compared the findings of Holter monitoring of children taking desipramine to nonmedicated children and found an association between desipramine plasma levels and single or paired premature atrial contractions, and runs of supraventricular tachycardia but concluded that these findings were clinically benign. Fletcher et al. (1993) reported that for 23 patients taking imipramine, cardiovascular function during controlled exercise did not induce supraventricular tachycardia or ventricular dysrhythmias. In this study, the mean plasma level of imipramine plus desipramine was 182 ng/ml, with a mean ratio of imipramine to desipramine of 0.7. Wagner and Fershtman (1993) reported an asymptomatic 12-year-old boy who developed significant prolongation of the QTc interval (0.45 sec) on 150 mg of desipramine per day that resolved with dose reduction to 125 mg per day. Studies are needed to investigate the effects of desipramine on cardiovascular function during and following controlled exercise. Werry (1994) has suggested that desipramine use be restricted to research protocols, while other authors call for further research and suggest judicious use of desipramine in appropriate patients (Ambrosini et al., 1994; Riddle, Geller, and Ryan, 1994). Patients with cardiovascular abnormalities, syncope, an abnormal electrocardiogram, or a family history of sudden death require further evaluation by a pediatric cardiologist prior to initiation of a tricyclic antidepressant (Riddle, Geller, and Ryan, 1993). Patients with healthy cardiovascular function should be monitored for cardiovascular function at baseline and with each increment in the dose of the tricyclic antidepressant.

Tricyclic Antidepressant-Induced Mania

Geller, Fox, and Fletcher (1993) reported on 54 children aged six to 12 years who were monitored for two to three years after treatment with nortriptyline for depression. Mania developed in nine out of 41 subjects who had received nortriptyline compared to none of the 13 subjects who had never taken a tricyclic antidepressant. Six of the nine subjects developed mania concurrent with nortriptyline administration. The authors acknowledge that it was not possible to separate nortriptyline-induced mania and mania that develops due to the natural course of illness. The authors indicate that there are more questions than answers concerning the use of the tricyclic antidepressants for children with depression, especially children with a family history of bipolar disorder. The authors encourage practitioners to monitor for signs and symptoms of mania or hypomania and to discontinue the tricyclic antidepressant as soon as possible.

Tricyclic-Induced Peripheral Neuropathy

Stept and Subramony (1988) reported a 14-year-old boy with hypothalamic disorder who developed a peripheral neuropathy while being treated with protriptyline for depression. The patient had numerous metabolic problems related to the hypothalamic disorder. The patient was taking protriptyline 20 mg at bedtime and methylphenidate 10 mg three times daily when he developed shuffling gait, decreased coordination, decreased strength in his lower extremities, and flat plantar reflexes. The patient's mother stated that the signs and symptoms had begun prior to the initiation of the methylphenidate, suggesting that the effects were due to the protriptyline. After discontinuation of the protriptyline, the patient recovered slowly over the next ten months. The authors acknowledge that the case is complicated by the metabolic abnormalities, but suggest that tricyclic antidepressants be used cautiously in patients with neural disease and metabolic abnormalities. Patients should be observed for signs and symptoms of peripheral neuropathy including paresthesias, weakness, and imbalance (Stept and Subramony, 1988).

Tricyclic-Induced Hyperpyrexia

Squires et al. (1992) reported on a 17-year-old boy who had been treated with 4.5 mg/kg/day of desipramine for approximately one year. After playing soccer for two hours on a humid day (95 degrees F) he became pale and weak and developed tonic-clonic seizure activity. Upon admission to the hospital, the patient had a core temperature of 108 degrees F, a pulse of 130 beats per minute, and blood pressure of 130/80 mm Hg. The patient's desipramine level was 85 mcg/ml. During the course of the 15-day hospitalization, the patient had massive diarrhea and low-grade, disseminated, intravascular clotting, with a marked increase in liver enzymes and serum creatinine. The patient's presentation resembled neuroleptic malignant syndrome (NMS), but lacked the typical muscular rigidity, autonomic instability, diaphoresis, and leukocytosis. The authors suggest that the tricyclic antidepressants induce a central nervous system imbalance in the ratio of norepinephrine to dopamine that may result in symptoms of NMS. The authors indicate that patients taking a tricyclic antidepressant should avoid strenuous exercise in extreme temperatures (Squires, 1992).

Tricyclic-Induced Hepatic Failure

Shaefer et al. (1990) reported the case of an 11-year-old, 41-kg boy who developed fulminant hepatic failure associated with the administration of imipramine 25 mg at bedtime for enuresis. The patient prior to taking imipramine was in good health and did not have a history of sickle cell disease, hepatitis, or cardiovascular disease. After taking the imipramine for seven days the patient became icteric, lethargic, anorexic, and complained of abdominal pain. Liver function tests showed a bilirubin (total/direct) of 15/7 mg/dl, aspartate aminotransferase (AST) 3860 IU/L, alanine aminotransferase (ALT) 3260 IU/L, and lactic dehydrogenase (LDH)of 837 IU/L. Laboratory evaluations for hepatitis, infectious mononucleosis, or sickle cell disease were negative. The patient over the next few days developed hepatic failure requiring liver transplant. The authors acknowledge that the exact mechanism of imipramine-induced hepatotoxicity is unknown; it may be related to a delayed hypersensitivity reaction, direct toxicity from imipramine or metabolites, or a combination of both.

DRUG INTERACTIONS

DRUG	DRUGS	EFFECT
TCA-D	Anticholinergic agents	Enhanced anticholinergic effect may occur resulting in confusion, hallucinations, delirium, CNS depression and other anticholinergic effects, constipation, blurred vision, tachycardia, urinary retention.
TCA-D	Antipsychotics, Pimozide	Increased anticholinergic, sedative, and cardiovascular effects. Both of these groups of medications may lower the seizure threshold, requiring adjustments in the dose or plasma levels of the anticonvulsants. The phenothiazines and the tricyclic antidepressants inhibit the hepatic metabolism of each other resulting in increased plasma levels of both drugs. Concurrent use of pimozide and TCA-D may result in cardiac arrhythmias, including prolongation of the QT interval on the electrocardiogram.
TCA-D	Barbiturates	Barbiturates may induce the metabolism of the TCA-D, resulting in lower TCA-D levels, and possibly higher levels of the secondary metabolites.
TCA-D	Cigarette smoking	Enhanced hepatic metabolism of the TCA-D potentially requiring higher doses of the TCA-D.
TCA-D	Carbamazepine	Carbamazepine may enhance the metabolism of the tricyclic antidepressants and may require increases in the dose of the tricyclic antidepressant (Brown et al., 1990). Carbamazepine-induced metabolism will increase the plasma levels of hydroxy metabolites of the tricyclic antidepressants. The hydroxy

metabolites are pharmacologically active and possibly cardiotoxic but are not routinely measured or reported with tricyclic antidepressant plasma levels. Increased monitoring for cardiovascular effects is suggested when the combination is used (Baldessarini et al., 1988; De la Fuente, 1992). The discontinuation of carbamazepine may result in higher TCA-D plasma levels.

TCA-D	Oral contraceptives, estrogens	Estrogens reduce the rate of metabolism, potentially resulting in higher blood levels of the TCA-D.
TCA-D	Monoamine oxidase inhibitors	Monoamine oxidase inhibitors must be discontinued two weeks prior to starting a TCA-D. Concurrent use has resulted in hypertensive crisis, convulsions, hyperpyrexia, and death, however, concurrent use has resulted in increased efficacy for patients that are nonresponsive or partially responsive to either drug. Both drugs should be initiated at low doses with gradual increases in the doses.
TCA-D	Fluoxetine	Fluoxetine may increase the plasma levels of the TCA-D. TCA-D dose reductions up to 50 percent may be required.
TCA-D	Beta blockers	Propranolol may inhibit the metabolism of the TCA-D and increase blood levels (Gillette and Tannery, 1994).
TCA-D	Methylphenidate	Methylphenidate will increase the plasma levels of the TCA-D by inhibiting hepatic metabolic enzymes. The adverse effects of nausea, dry mouth, tremor, headaches, anorexia, and tiredness may increase if the combination is used (Pataki et al., 1993). Although combinations of methylphenidate and imipramine have been used successfully, they have resulted in confusion, marked aggression, and severe agitation, even psychosis (Grob and Coyle, 1986).

TCA-D	Sympathomimetics, beta-agonists	Concurrent use may result in increased heart rate, blood pressure, and arrhthymias.
TCA-D	Thyroid hormones	Concurrent use may result in increased therapeutic and toxic effects of both medications. Toxic effects include cardiac arrhythmias and CNS stimulation.
TCA-D	Antihistamines, terfenadine, astemazole	Concurrent use can prolong the QT corrected intervals on the electrocardiogram, resulting in Torsade de Pointes, a life-threatening ventricular tachyrhythmia (Diamond, 1993).
TCA-D	Cimetidine	Cimetidine is an inhibitor of the cytochrome P450 enzyme system. Cimetidine inhibits the metabolism of the TCA-D resulting in higher TCA-D plasma levels.
TCA-D	Clonidine	Concurrent use has resulted in increased blood pressure. Concurrent use is not recommended.
TCA-D	Alcohol, CNS depressants	Concurrent use may increase the central nervous system (CNS) effects, respiratory depression, and hypotensive effects. The use of alcohol is contraindicated.

MONITORING GUIDELINES

Baseline Assessment:

- History and physical, including weight and height of the patient.
- Blood pressure and pulse, electrocardiogram (EKG), and family history of sudden death or cardiovascular disease. Patients with congenital or acquired cardiac disease, murmur, pathologic rhythm disturbances, family history of sudden death or cardiomyopathy, diastolic hypertension, or questionable cardiac status should have further cardiac evaluation before a tricyclic antidepressant is initiated. Further cardiac evaluation includes a 24-hour

Holter monitor and an echocardiographic evaluation (Biederman et al., 1989b). Patients who have pretreatment EKG abnormalities or cardiac disease are more likely to develop PR interval prolongation (Bartels et al., 1991).

- Observe the patient for involuntary movements or tics.
- Thyroid function tests, serum protein, albumin, bilirubin direct and indirect, alkaline phosphatase, serum glutamic oxaloacetic transaminase (SGOT), serum glutamic pyruvic transaminase (SGPT), lactic dehydrogenase (LDH), creatinine phosphokinase (CPK), and EEG if there is a patient or family history of seizures or abnormal EEG. Other laboratory tests as indicated.
- For patients treated for enuresis, rule out all other causes of enuresis including neurological/spinal abnormalities, diabetes insipidus or mellitus, chronic renal failure, and bacteriuria. Check urine for specific gravity, glucose, protein, blood, and infection (Friman and Warzak, 1990). In addition, rule out drugs known to cause or exacerbate enuresis, e.g., lithium or antipsychotics.

Time Pattern for Response:

- In the treatment of enuresis, response may occur the first night, but usually is evident within the first week of therapy. For attention-deficit/hyperactivity disorder, the effects have been reported to occur within the first week, but may require up to four weeks of treatment. Obsessive compulsive disorder requires three or more weeks of treatment to see a response. Efficacy has not been proven in the treatment of depression, but anti-depressant effects in adults are noted within three weeks of treatment.

Follow-Up Assessment:

- Weight and height of the patient should be obtained at three to six month intervals.
- Blood pressure and pulse should routinely be obtained during dose titration and during follow-up. For children less than ten years of age, reduce the dose or discontinue

the medication if the resting heart rate is greater than 110 beats/minute, or if the resting blood pressure is greater than 140/90 or persistently greater than 130/85. For children over ten years of age, reduce the dose or discontinue the medication if the resting heart rate is greater than 100 beats per minute, or if the resting blood pressure is greater than 150/95 or persistently greater than 140/85 (Ryan, 1992).

- Electrocardiogram should be obtained after each dose increase and after reaching steady-state blood levels. For children and adolescents, reduce the dose or discontinue the medication if the corrected QT interval (QTc) is greater than 0.45 seconds (Riddle et al., 1991; Tingelstad, 1991), or if the QRS interval is greater than 0.12 seconds or widens more than 50 percent over the baseline QRS interval (Ryan, 1992). In addition, for children less than ten years of age, reduce the dose or discontinue the medication if the PR interval is greater than 0.18 seconds. For children ten years of age and older, reduce the dose or discontinue the medication if the PR interval is greater than 0.20 seconds (Ryan, 1992).
- Liver function tests should be obtained according to patient status. Nausea, anorexia, fever, and myalgias may be signs of drug-induced hepatitis.
- Observe the patient for involuntary movements or tics.
- Tricyclic antidepressant plasma levels may be used as a guide to therapy. Patients who are not responding to therapy may have a low plasma level that requires an increase in dose to achieve efficacy. Patients who are having numerous side effects at a low dose may have a high plasma level requiring a dose reduction.
- Complete blood count according to patient status and for patients with fever, sore throat or other infections, unusual bleeding or bruising.
- For patients with epilepsy, the tricyclic antidepressants may lower the seizure threshold requiring adjustments in the plasma concentrations of the anticonvulsants needed

to control seizure activity. Monitoring for seizure activity and plasma levels is suggested.

- Monitor for proper use of the tricyclic antidepressants. Assess the risk of TCA-D overdose due to accidental overdose or intentional suicide gestures or attempts.

Drug Discontinuation:

- Abrupt withdrawal is not recommended. Rapid withdrawal may result in flu-like symptoms such as nausea, vomiting, abdominal pain, drowsiness/fatigue, diminished appetite, tearfulness, apathy/withdrawal, and headache (Law, Petti, and Kazdin, 1981). A tricyclic antidepressant should be withdrawn over a one- to three-week period or according to the patient's ability to tolerate the withdrawal process. If withdrawal symptoms develop, restart the medication or increase the dose and decrease the rate of tapering according to the patient's status.

SPECIAL INSTRUCTIONS FOR PARENTS/CARE GIVERS/ CHILDREN/ADOLESCENTS

- The tricyclic antidepressants may be toxic if too much medication is taken. Administer only the prescribed dose. Children may want to take extra doses to increase response. Do not double doses. Keep this medication locked away from the patient and other children and adolescents.
- Tricyclic antidepressants may cause drowsiness during the first few weeks. If this happens, the child should not participate in activities that require alertness, such as riding a bike or driving a car.
- Dry mouth is a common side effect of the tricyclic antidepressants. Drinking sips of water, sucking on crushed ice, chewing sugarless gum, or sucking on hard candy will help with this side effect. Encourage regular brushing of the teeth.
- The tricyclic antidepressants may cause constipation. Encourage the patient to exercise, drink plenty of fluids, and eat fruits, vegetables, and fiber-containing foods to help with

constipation. If necessary a mild stool softener, such as docusate sodium, may be used daily to relieve constipation. Docusate sodium is an nonprescription medication; ask your pharmacist or physician to suggest the proper dose and frequency.

- The patient may need to have blood drawn to determine the amount of drug in the blood. The blood is drawn in the morning, before taking the morning dose.

- The effects of the medication on the heart and blood pressure will be monitored with blood pressure checks and electrocardiograms. If the patient's heartbeat gets very fast, call the physician right away. This medication can cause dizziness when standing up too quickly. Instruct the patient to rise slowly during the first few weeks of therapy. Dizziness will go away after a few weeks of taking the medication.

- The tricyclic antidepressants will increase sensitivity to the sun. The patient should wear a sunscreen lotion on exposed skin and protective clothing, including a hat to prevent severe sunburn. In addition, overheating can occur; patients should be encouraged to exercise in moderation, take frequent breaks, and drink plenty of water.

- The tricyclic antidepressants may cause the following serious side effects: hyperactivity, insomnia, seizures or convulsions, hallucinations (hearing voices or seeing things that are not there), nausea, loss of appetite, fever, muscle pain, or other unusual behaviors or effects. Call the physician right away if any of these side effects occur. Although many children have a good response to desipramine, unexplained sudden deaths in children taking desipramine have occurred.

- Other side effects of the medication that need to be reported to your physician include: high or low blood pressure, trouble urinating, blurred vision, muscle twitches, weight gain or loss, appetite changes, tiredness, and irritability.

- In the treatment of enuresis, be sure to have the child empty their bladder prior to bedtime.

- Be sure to tell any physicians, pharmacists, and dentists that this medication is being taken.

- Avoid the use of alcoholic beverages during therapy with this medication, including cough, cold, and flu products that contain alcohol.
- Do not use any other medications without consulting your physician or pharmacist.
- Do not stop taking this medication suddenly, without checking with your physician. The physician will want to decrease the dose slowly over a few weeks, before stopping completely.

PRODUCTS AVAILABLE

Amitriptyline is available as Elavil® from Stuart Pharmaceuticals and as Endep® form Roche Laboratories. Amitriptyline is also available in generic form. All Elavil® tablets are film-coated and non-scored. Elavil® 10 mg is blue, round, and imprinted with Stuart 40. Elavil® 25 mg is yellow, round, and imprinted with Stuart 45. Elavil® 50 mg is beige, round, and imprinted with Stuart 41. Elavil® 100 mg is mauve, round, and imprinted with Stuart 43. Elavil® 150 mg is blue, capsule shaped, and imprinted with Stuart 47. All Endep® tablets are film-coated, scored, and imprinted with Roche. Endep® 10 mg, 25 mg, and 50 mg are all orange in color, and imprinted with Endep 10, Endep 25, and Endep 50, respectively. Endep® 100 mg is peach, and imprinted with Endep 100. Endep® 150 mg is salmon, and imprinted with Endep 150.

Clomipramine is available as Anafranil® from Ciba Geigy Pharmaceuticals. Anafranil® 25 mg is an ivory/melon yellow capsule imprinted with Anafranil 25 mg. Anafranil® 50 mg is an ivory/aqua blue capsule imprinted with Anafranil 50 mg. Anafranil® 75 mg is an ivory/yellow capsule imprinted with Anafranil 75 mg.

Desipramine is available as Norpramin® from Marion Merrell Dow and is available in generic form. Norpramin® 10 mg is a blue tablet imprinted with 68-7. Norpramin® 25 mg is a yellow tablet imprinted with Norpramin 25. Norpramin® 50 mg is a green tablet imprinted with Norpramin 50. Norpramin® 75 mg is an orange tablet imprinted with Norpramin 75. Norpramin® 100 mg is a peach tablet imprinted with Norpramin 100. Norpramin® 150 mg is a white tablet imprinted with Norpramin 150.

Imipramine is available as Janimine® from Abbott Laboratories, as Tofranil® from Ciba Geigy Pharmaceuticals, and is available in generic form. Janimine® 50 mg is a peach, oval, film-coated tablet, and contains tartrazine. Tofranil® 10 mg is a coral, triangular tablet imprinted with Geigy 32. Tofranil® 25 mg is a coral, round tablet imprinted with Geigy 140. Tofranil® 50 mg is a coral, round, tablet imprinted with Geigy 136. Tofranil PM® 75 mg is a coral capsule imprinted with Geigy 20. Tofranil PM® 125 mg is a dark yellow/coral capsule imprinted with Geigy 40. Tofranil PM® 150 mg is a coral capsule imprinted with Geigy 22.

Nortriptyline is available as Aventyl® from Eli Lilly, as Pamelor® from Sandoz Pharmaceuticals, and is available in generic form. Aventyl® 10 mg is a white and yellow capsule imprinted with Lilly H 17. Aventyl® 25 mg is a white and yellow capsule imprinted with Lilly H 19. Aventyl® liquid contains 10 mg per 5 ml and contains 4 percent alcohol. Pamelor® 10 mg is an orange and white capsule imprinted with Pamelor 10 mg, Sandoz. Pamelor® 25 mg is an orange and white capsule imprinted with Pamelor 25 mg, Sandoz. Pamelor® 50 mg is a white capsule imprinted with Pamelor 50 mg, Sandoz. Pamelor® 75 mg is an orange capsule imprinted with Pamelor 75 mg, Sandoz. Pamelor® solution contains 10 mg per 5 ml with a 4 percent alcohol content.

COST

GENERIC NAME	TRADENAME	AWP*	AWP* per dose
Amitriptyline 10 mg		$1.43 for 100 tablets	$0.02 per tablet
Amitriptyline 25 mg		$1.65 for 100 tablets	$0.02 per tablet
Amitriptyline 50 mg		$2.40 for 100 tablets	$0.03 per tablet

Amitriptyline 100 mg		$3.38 for 100 tablets	$0.04 per tablet
Amitriptyline 150 mg		$7.05 for 100 tablets	$0.08 per tablet
Amitriptyline	Elavil® 10 mg	$17.87 for 100 tablets	$0.18 per tablet
	Elavil® 25 mg	$35.83 for 100 tablets	$0.36 per tablet
	Elavil® 50 mg	$63.73 for 100 tablets	$0.64 per tablet
	Elavil® 100 mg	$110.34 for 100 tablets	$1.10 per tablet
	Elavil® 150 mg	$157.01 for 100 tablets	$1.58 per tablet
Amitriptyline	Endep® 10 mg	$15.08 for 100 tablets	$0.16 per tablet
	Endep® 25 mg	$29.82 for 100 tablets	$0.30 per tablet
	Endep® 50 mg	$52.99 for 100 tablets	$0.53 per tablet
	Endep® 100 mg	$96.27 for 100 tablets	$0.97 per tablet
	Endep® 150 mg	$147.86 for 100 tablets	$1.48 per tablet
Clomipramine	Anafranil® 25 mg	$76.01 for 100 capsules	$0.77 per capsule
	Anafranil® 50 mg	$102.50 for 100 capsules	$1.03 per capsule
	Anafranil® 75 mg	$134.92 for 100 capsules	$1.35 per capsule
Desipramine 10 mg		$15.29 for 100 tablets	$0.15 per tablet
Desipramine 25 mg		$9.53 for 100 tablets	$0.10 per tablet
Desipramine 50 mg		$14.93 for 100 tablets	$0.15 per tablet
Desipramine 75 mg		$18.38 for 100 tablets	$0.19 per tablet
Desipramine 100 mg		$43.53 for 100 tablets	$0.44 per tablet
Desipramine 150 mg		$59.80 for 100 tablets	$0.60 per tablet
Desipramine	Norpramin® 10 mg	$47.58 for 100 tablets	$0.48 per tablet
	Norpramin® 25 mg	$57.18 for 100 tablets	$0.58 per tablet
	Norpramin® 50 mg	$107.46 for 100 tablets	$1.08 per tablet
	Norpramin® 75 mg	$136.80 for 100 tablets	$1.37 per tablet
	Norpramin® 100 mg	$179.70 for 100 tablets	$1.80 per tablet
	Norpramin® 150 mg	$260.40 for 100 tablets	$2.61 per tablet
Imipramine 10 mg		$1.83 for 100 tablets	$0.02 per tablet
Imipramine 25 mg		$2.33 for 100 tablets	$0.03 per tablet
Imipramine 50 mg		$3.08 for 100 tablets	$0.04 per tablet
Imipramine	Janimine® 50 mg	$9.22 for 100 tablets	$0.10 per tablet
Imipramine	Tofranil® 10 mg	$25.33 for 100 tablets	$0.26 per tablet
	Tofranil® 25 mg	$42.36 for 100 tablets	$0.43 per tablet
	Tofranil® 50 mg	$71.96 for 100 tablets	$0.72 per tablet
	Tofranil PM® 75 mg	$100.65 for 100 capsules	$1.01 per capsule
	Tofranil PM® 125 mg	$132.32 for 100 capsules	$1.33 per capsule
	Tofranil PM® 150 mg	$188.09 for 100 capsules	$1.89 per capsule
Nortriptyline 10 mg		$35.10 for 100 capsules	$0.36 per capsule
Nortriptyline 25 mg		$70.18 for 100 capsules	$0.71 per capsule

Nortriptyline 50 mg		$131.83 for 100 capsules	$1.32 per capsule
Nortriptyline 75 mg		$200.99 for 100 capsules	$2.01 per capsule
Nortriptyline	Aventyl® 10 mg	$41.69 for 100 capsules	$0.42 per capsule
	Aventyl® 25 mg	$83.24 for 100 capsules	$0.84 per capsule
	Aventyl® liquid (10 mg per 5 ml)	$45.83 for 500 ml	$0.46 per 5 ml
Nortriptyline	Pamelor® 10 mg	$42.96 for 100 capsules	$0.43 per capsule
	Pamelor® 25 mg	$85.86 for 100 capsules	$0.86 per capsule
	Pamelor® 50 mg	$161.88 for 100 capsules	$1.62 per capsule
	Pamelor® 75 mg	$246.84 for 100 capsules	$2.47 per capsule
	Pamelor® solution (10 mg per 5 ml)	$51.38 for 500 ml	$0.52 per 5 ml

* AWP is the average wholesale price to the pharmacist that is listed in the *1994 Redbook* (Cardinale, 1994).

BUPROPION

Bupropion hydrochloride

Wellbutrin® is marketed by Burroughs Wellcome.

DSM-IV INDICATIONS

Attention-Deficit/Hyperactivity Disorder (??)

> FDA: Not approved for use in children less than 18 years old (*PDR*, 1994).
> USP: Safety and efficacy have not been established (*USPDI*, 1994).

CONTRAINDICATIONS: Hypersensitivity to bupropion; patients with seizure disorders or patients who are at risk of developing seizures (*see* Adverse Effects); patients with a current or prior diagnosis of bulimia or anorexia nervosa due to the increased risk of seizures (Horne et al., 1988); concurrent administration with a monoamine oxidase inhibitor (*see* Drug Interactions).

PHARMACOLOGY: Bupropion is an antidepressant of the aminoketone class and is chemically unrelated to the tricyclic antidepressants and other available antidepressants. The structure of bupropion resembles that of diethylpropion, an amphetamine congener. The mechanism of action of bupropion is unknown. Bupropion does not inhibit the monoamine oxidase enzyme and is a weak blocker of neuronal uptake of serotonin, norepinephrine, and dopamine. Bupropion may also have weak dopamine agonist activity. Bupropion may induce its own metabolism suggesting that the pharmacological effect of bupropion and its metabolites may be altered with chronic use.

STUDIES OF BUPROPION EFFICACY

Attention-Deficit/Hyperactivity Disorder (ADHD)

Simeon, Ferguson, and Van Wyck Fleet (1986) reported an open clinical trial of 17 boys (seven to 13 years old) who were treated with bupropion for attention-deficit disorder with hyperactivity and/or conduct disorder. Exclusion criteria for this study included seizure disorders, mental retardation, or any significant medical condition. Each patient was given placebo for four weeks to identify placebo responders. Bupropion was administered over eight weeks with initial doses of 50 mg per day for the first week, 50 mg two times daily for the second week, and then 50 mg three times daily for the remainder of the trial. Two weeks of placebo were then given to determine withdrawal effects of bupropion, or relapse. Five patients had marked clinical global improvement, seven had moderate improvement, two had mild improvement, and three had no improvement. The symptoms that were reported to be most improved were hyperactivity, conduct, affect, anxiety, and sleep. Bupropion was less effective in improving attention span, distractibility, and impulsivity. Adverse effects were assessed in this study, and increased appetite and nausea/vomiting occurred more frequently with bupropion than placebo. There were no reported changes in blood pressure, pulse, or EKG findings. Thirteen of 17 patients showed decreases in body weight during bupropion therapy. The authors recommended that double-blind studies be conducted (Simeon, Ferguson, and Van Wyck Fleet, 1986).

Casat, Pleasants, and Van Wyck Fleet (1987) reported a four-week double-blind trial of 31 children (six to 12 years old) with attention-deficit disorder with hyperactivity. Exclusion criteria included the above criteria from the Simeon study in addition to evidence of a tic disorder. Bupropion 3 mg/kg to a maximum of 6 mg/kg were administered in two divided daily doses. Patient improvement was noted on the teachers' assessment of hyperactivity and on the Clinical Global Impression scale. The parents' assessment of hyperactivity and the teachers' assessment of conduct showed no improvement with bupropion. Adverse effects in one child included rash, perioral edema, and agitation after 18 days of bupropion therapy. The authors report no changes in heart rate, blood pressure, height, weight, prolactin levels, laboratory values, EEG, or EKG (Casat, Ferguson, and Van Wyck Fleet, 1987).

Clay et al. (1988) reported a four-week double-blind placebo controlled trial of 28 prepubertal children (six to 12 years old) with attention-deficit disorder with hyperactivity. Exclusion criteria were history of seizures or head trauma, or an IQ less than 70. Patients were assigned a placebo or bupropion in a 1:2 ratio respectively. The dosage of bupropion was initiated at 3 mg/kg/day and titrated to an optimum dose at day 21 of the trial. Optimal doses of bupropion ranged from 3.1 to 7.1 mg/kg up to 250 mg per day. The mean dose of bupropion was 5.3 mg/kg. Two patients developed a rash while on bupropion, but no patient developed tics, seizures, or a psychotic reaction. Children who were given bupropion showed more improvement on the Clinical Global Impression scales for Improvement and Severity than children who were given placebo. There was a trend for improvement with bupropion for the hyperactivity scores. The authors note that the results of this study are compounded by the differences between the bupropion and placebo subjects at baseline. They also noted their impression that children with ADHD, with prominent symptoms of conduct disorder, responded better to bupropion (Clay et al., 1988).

Studies of bupropion in the treatment of attention-deficit/hyperactivity disorder are limited by the small number of subjects and the short time periods of investigation. The research exclusion criteria of history of seizures or previous head trauma, tic disorders, and any significant medical condition is applicable to clinical practice. Additional exclusions from bupropion therapy, including a history of bulimia, are listed in the contraindications section above.

DEVELOPMENTAL PHARMACOKINETICS

Absorption: Rapidly absorbed from the gastrointestinal tract.

Biotransformation: Bupropion is extensively metabolized to active and inactive metabolites. Bupropion undergoes an extensive first-pass effect and only a small portion of any oral dose reaches the systemic circulation intact. Four basic metabolites of bupropion have been identified: the erythro-amino alcohol, the threo-amino alcohol, erythro-amino diol, and a morpholinol metabolite. The morpholinol metabolite appears in the systemic circulation almost as rapidly as the parent drug and is half as potent as bupropion in animal tests. The peak level of the morpholinol metabolite is three times the level of the parent drug and has a half-life of 24 hours. The clinical significance of these metabolites for children is unknown.

Onset of action: The onset of action for attention-deficit/hyperactivity disorder is not known. Antidepressant effect occurs in three to four weeks in adults.

Time to peak effect/serum concentration: In adults, the peak plasma concentration is achieved within two to three hours

Duration of action: Approximately six to eight hours for children (Burroughs Wellcome, personal communication).

Distribution: In adults, bupropion is 75 to 85 percent bound to human albumin at levels up to 200 mcg/ml.

Half-life: In adults, the average half-life is 14 hours (range eight to 24 hours).

Plasma/saliva levels: Therapeutic levels have not been established. There is a substantial variability in trough levels of bupropion and metabolites. In addition, the steady-state plasma levels of the metabolites were ten to 100 times the concentration of the parent drug.

DOSAGE RANGES

Attention-Deficit/Hyperactivity Disorder

Investigation studies have used oral doses of 3 to 6 mg/kg/day, to a maximum of 25 mg/day. The total daily dose is administered throughout the day in three evenly divided doses. Insomnia may be avoided by avoiding bedtime doses. Gradual increases in dose are recommended to minimize agitation, motor restlessness, and insomnia during the first few days of treatment. Unfortunately, the dose should be according to the marketed tablet size of 75 or 100 mg. Splitting of the tablets is difficult due to the surface coating on the non-scored tablets. A sustained release product is under development and will include a 50 mg dose. Bupropion is not stable in solution (Burroughs Wellcome, personal communication).

ADVERSE EFFECTS REPORTED IN CHILDREN AND ADOLESCENTS

COMMON

The adverse effects that have been found in the investigations (listed above) in children and adolescents are increased appetite, nausea, vomiting, decreases in body weight, rash, perioral edema, and agitation. In addition, for children with attention-deficit/hyperactivity disorder and Tourette's syndrome bupropion may exacerbate tics (Spencer et al., 1993). One case report described a child who developed hypomania (*see also* Adverse Reactions/ Case Reports). The findings in the adult population include increased restlessness, agitation, anxiety, confusion and insomnia, dry mouth, headache, nausea/vomiting, rashes, constipation, anorexia, dizziness, increased sweating, tremor, and weight loss.

LESS COMMON

Seizures: There are several risk factors that may predispose a patient to develop seizures while taking bupropion: history of seizures (including febrile convulsions), structural abnormalities of the central nervous system, sedative/ hypnotic withdrawal including alcohol detoxification, concurrent use of drugs that lower the seizure threshold (*see* Drug Interactions), high dose, improper administration/not giving in divided daily doses, recent or rapid escalation of bupropion, a history or presence of anorexia or bulimia nervosa, overdose, known EEG abnormality, and high plasma levels of the bupropion or metabolites (Davidson, 1989; Johnston et al., 1991). In addition to seizures, other CNS reactions include hypomania, delusions, hallucinations, psychotic episodes, euphoria, and paranoia.

ALLERGIC REACTION: In several investigations, patients have developed a rash that subsided after discontinuation of bupropion.

TOXICITY: Possible seizure activity, overstimulation, excitement.

ADVERSE REACTIONS/CASE REPORTS

Tics

Spencer et al. (1993) reported a series of four children with attention-deficit/hyperactivity disorder and Tourette's syndrome. Each of the children had been previously treated with stimulants that exacerbated the tics. For various reasons a trial of bupropion was initiated. After two to eight weeks of bupropion therapy, the patients manifested a worsening of their tics. Upon discontinuation of the bupropion, the tics improved to their baseline level. The authors discuss the dopaminergic mechanism of the pathophysiology of tics, and point out that bupropion is chemically related to the CNS stimulants and may have a weak dopaminergic effect. Whether bupropion or the stimulants will cause the earlier expression of tics in a patient predisposed to tics or Tourette's syndrome remains controversial (Spencer et al., 1993).

Hypomania

Bloomingdale (1990) reported a 12-year-old, 40-kg boy with attention-deficit/hyperactivity disorder and opposition behavior that had been treated with methylphenidate, and magnesium pemoline and clonidine. Therapy with methylphenidate was associated with severe headaches, so magnesium pemoline and clonidine were initiated. While on this therapy the patient developed a repetitive clearing of his throat which was considered to be tic-like. Bupropion was substituted for the magnesium pemoline and the clonidine was continued. Up to 275 mg of bupropion was prescribed in three divided doses. After an unspecified time the patient manifested hypomanic symptoms, and the dose of bupropion was reduced. The duration of therapy or whether the child developed tics on bupropion was not reported (Bloomingdale, 1990).

DRUG INTERACTIONS

DRUG	DRUGS	EFFECT
Bupropion	Alcohol	The concurrent use or discontinuation of alcohol may increase the likelihood of seizures.
Bupropion	Benzodiazepines	Abrupt withdrawal of benzodiazepines may precipitate seizures.
Bupropion	Antipsychotics, Antidepressants, Lithium	Concurrent use of these agents may lower the seizure threshold and increase the likelihood of seizures.
Bupropion	Monoamine oxidase inhibitors	Concurrent use of bupropion and these agents may increase the acute toxicity of bupropion and is contraindicated. A two-week drug-free interval is recommended between discontinuation of a monoamine oxidase inhibitor and initiation of bupropion.
Bupropion	Hepatic enzyme inducers	Bupropion may also be an enzyme inducer in humans and may contribute to enzyme induction from concurrently administered drugs. The increased metabolism of bupropion or the other drugs may occur. Examples include; barbiturates, carbamazepine, griseofulvin, phenytoin, primidone, and rifampin.
Bupropion	Hepatic enzyme inhibitors	The metabolism of bupropion may be inhibited by these drugs, resulting in higher serum levels and possible increase in the risk of seizures. Examples include: cimetidine, oral contraceptives, diltiazem, disulfiram, divalproex, erythromycin, fluconazole, fluoroquinolones, isoniazid, ketoconazole, itraconazole, metoprolol, miconazole, omeprazole, propranolol, valproic acid, and verapamil.

MONITORING GUIDELINES

Baseline Assessment:

- History and physical, including height and weight of the patient.
- Determine history of seizures or head trauma (electroencephalogram, if questionable).
- Assess compliance for a multiple daily dosing regimen.
- Determine recent medication history for possible drug interactions.

Time Patterns for Response: Unknown in children with ADHD.

Follow-Up Assessment:

- Height and weight, according to patient status.
- Monitor for therapeutic effect and adverse effects. Include a neurological check for tics.
- Laboratory workup: according to patient status.

Drug Discontinuation: According to patient status.

SPECIAL INSTRUCTIONS FOR PARENTS/CARE GIVERS/ CHILDREN/ADOLESCENTS

- Administer bupropion in equally divided doses three or four times daily to minimize the risk of seizures.
- Do not double doses.
- Avoid the use of alcohol.
- Do not take more or less medication than prescribed.
- Bupropion may be taken with food to lessen stomach upset.
- Store this medication and all medications away from the patient and other children and adolescents.
- Do not give your child any other medications without consulting your physician or pharmacist.

PRODUCTS AVAILABLE

Bupropion is marketed as Wellbutrin® from Burroughs Well-come. Wellbutrin® is available in a 75 mg yellow-gold, round, non-scored, biconvex tablet imprinted with Wellbutrin 75. Wellbutrin® is also available in a 100 mg red, round, biconvex, non-scored tablet imprinted with Wellbutrin 100.

COST

GENERIC NAME	TRADENAME	AWP*	AWP* per dose
Bupropion	Wellbutrin® 75 mg	$55.00 for 100 tablets	$0.55 per tablet
	Wellbutrin® 100 mg	$73.00 for 100 tablets	$0.73 per tablet

* AWP is the average wholesale price to the pharmacist that is listed in the *1994 Redbook* (Cardinale, 1994).

MONOAMINE OXIDASE INHIBITORS

Phenelzine

Nardil® is marketed by Parke-Davis.

Tranylcypromine

Parnate® is marketed by SmithKline Beecham Pharmaceuticals.

DSM-IV INDICATIONS

Depression, treatment resistant (???)
Attention-Deficit/Hyperactivity Disorder, treatment resistant (???)

FDA: Safety and efficacy have not been established in pediatric populations (*PDR,* 1994).
USP: Safety and efficacy have not been established in pediatric populations (*USPDI,* 1994).

CONTRAINDICATIONS: Hypersensitivity to any monoamine oxidase inhibitor; inability to follow the diet and drug restrictions; children or adolescents who are impulsive or have a history of substance abuse, alcoholism; pregnancy; concurrent use of sympathomimetics, meperidine, or other psychotropic medications; renal or hepatic impairment; congestive heart failure, cardiovascular disease; pheochromocytoma; asthma; diabetes mellitus; epilepsy; frequent or severe headaches; or hyperthyroidism.

PHARMACOLOGY: Monoamine oxidase is an enzyme that metabolizes biogenic amines. Monoamine oxidase inhibitors (MAO-I) increase the concentrations of serotonin, norepinephrine, and dopamine in the central nervous system by inhibiting the activity of the monoamine oxidase enzyme. The nonspecific monoamine oxidase inhibitors, phenelzine and tranylcypromine, inhibit both subtypes of the monoamine oxidase enzyme, A and B. Phenelzine and tranylcypromine also down-regulate (desensitize) alpha-2 or bet-adrenergic and serotonin receptors. Down-regulation of these receptors is correlated with antidepressant activity. The monoamine oxidase inhibitors also prevent the inactivation of tyramine by hepatic and gastrointestinal monoamine oxidase. Increases in tyramine result in the release of norepinephrine from the sympathetic nerve terminals and result in an increase in blood pressure. Patients who take monoamine oxidase inhibitors must maintain a low-tyramine diet.

In addition, there are numerous drug interactions with monoamine oxidase inhibitors. There is minimal information on the use of the monoamine oxidase inhibitors in children or adolescents, and practitioners are encouraged to be familiar with all the potential hazards associated with their use.

STUDIES OF MONOAMINE OXIDASE INHIBITOR EFFICACY

Attention-Deficit/Hyperactivity Disorder

Zametkin et al. (1985) reported a double-blind, crossover trial in 14 boys (aged eight to 12 years) with attention-deficit disorder. Each patient received a two-week placebo washout phase which was followed by two, four-week drug periods. Each drug period was separated by a two-week placebo washout. All patients received dextroamphetamine (10 mg in the morning and 5 mg at noon) during one of the active drug phases. Six children received clorgyline and eight received tranylcypromine (5 mg in the morning and 5 mg at noon) during the other active drug phase. After six children had completed the protocol on clorgyline, the drug became unavailable and the study continued with tranylcypromine. MAO-I therapy resulted in a significant and rapid reduction in ADHD symptoms with minimal adverse effects. The authors report that MAO-I therapy in this study is comparable to dextroamphetamine therapy (Zametkin et al., 1985).

Depression

Ryan et al. (1988) reported a retrospective chart review of 23 adolescents (aged 11 to 18 years) who were treated with monoamine oxidase inhibitors (MAO-I) for tricyclic antidepressant-resistant depression. Fourteen of the patients had concurrent diagnoses of major depression superimposed on dysthymia, atypical depression, psychotic depression, bipolar II disorder, anxiety disorder, and conduct disorder. Patients were treated with a combination of a different tricyclic antidepressant and either tranylcypromine or phenelzine. Adverse effects were reported while on the tricyclic antidepressant (TCA-D), and after the addition of the MAO-I. Side effects that were increased while on the MAO-I augmentation therapy include urinary retention, orthostatic hypotension, palpitations, blurred vision, peripheral weakness, insomnia, and headaches.

One patient upon withdrawal of tranylcypromine had frequent nightmares for two weeks. Dietary noncompliance, both accidental and deliberate, were common. Seven of the patients were noncompliant with the diet; two of them had significant symptoms. One patient had headaches and hypertension that was treated with chlorpromazine, and he suffered no residual effects. Another patient developed myoclonic jerks that resolved without residual effects. Two patients developed brief hypomanic effects with on a TCA-D and MAO-I, but continued with the therapy. One patient developed a mixed manic-depressive picture with predominantly irritable, not euphoric mood. Overall 11 out of 23 patients had a good clinical response to the TCA-D and MAO-I combination with good dietary compliance. The authors suggest that for patients who are impulsive, unreliable, or who have unreliable families, the risks of MAO-I therapy may outweigh the benefits. The authors also suggest the MAO-I augmentation therapy may be indicated in TCA-D resistant depression in selected adolescents (Ryan et al., 1988).

DEVELOPMENTAL PHARMACOKINETICS

Absorption: Phenelzine and tranylcypromine are well absorbed orally.

Onset of action: Zametkin et al. (1985) reported that the onset of action of tranylcypromine in the treatment of ADHD was immediate and comparable to the onset of dextroamphetamine.

Time to peak effect: Unknown.

Duration of action: The duration of activity of the MAO-I has not been studied in the pediatric population; however, in adults the clinical effect of phenelzine may continue for two weeks after discontinuation. The effects of tranylcypromine in adults may continue up to ten days following discontinuation.

DOSAGE RANGES

Attention-Deficit/Hyperactivity Disorder

In the study reported by Zametkin et al. (1985) the doses administered to the eight children who received tranylcypromine in the treatment of ADHD were 5 mg in the morning and 5 mg at noon. There are no further dosing recommendations available.

Depression

In the MAO-I augmentation study by Ryan et al. (1988), the doses administered were not reported, with the exception of the children who were noncompliant with the low tyramine diet. For adults, tranylcypromine is dosed between 10 and 60 mg per day. Tranylcypromine 30 mg per day administered in divided doses is a typical adult dose. In adults, phenelzine is initiated at 15 mg three times a day and increased up to a maximum of 90 mg per day.

ADVERSE EFFECTS REPORTED IN CHILDREN AND ADOLESCENTS

COMMON

> Preliminary short-term investigations (Ryan et al., 1988; Zametkin et al., 1985) report side effects of feeling tired, sleepiness, decreased appetite, insomnia, headache, urinary retention, orthostatic hypotension, palpitations, blurred vision, peripheral weakness, and hypomania (*see* Less Common Adverse Effects).

LESS COMMON

Due to the lack of studies, there is a lack of information in this area. Until further information is available, practitioners are encouraged to monitor for the adverse effects that have been reported in adults.

ALLERGIC REACTION: Skin rashes have been reported in adults. The incidence of allergic reactions to the MAO-I is unknown in children, but appears to be low in adults.

TOXICITY: Hypertensive crisis may result from the accidental or purposeful ingestion of restricted foods or drugs. In adults, the signs and symptoms of hypertensive crisis include headache, palpitations, neck stiffness or soreness, nausea, vomiting, sweating, cold clammy skin, dilated pupils, photophobia, tachycardia, bradycardia, or chest pain. Ryan et al. (1988) reported one 16-year-old male, treated with tranylcypromine 40 mg/day, who ate a sausage and subsequently developed a headache and a blood pressure reading of 162/104. This patient was treated with chlorpromazine and recovered without residual effects. Treatment of hypertensive crisis in children and adolescents has not been investigated.

DRUG INTERACTIONS

DRUG	DRUGS	EFFECT
MAO-I	Tricyclic Antidepressants (TCA-D), MAO-I, Bupropion, Fluoxetine, Cyclobenzaprine, Carbamazepine	A TCA-D should not be added to MAO-I therapy. An MAO-I must be discontinued for two weeks prior to the initiation of a bupropion, or an MAO-I. The addition of an MAO-I to current TCA-D therapy has been reported (Ryan et al., 1988). To avoid serious adverse effects including death, fluoxetine must be discontinued five weeks prior to the initiation of an MAO-I. An

		MAO-I should be discontinued for two weeks prior to the initiation of fluoxetine. Cyclobenzaprine and carbamazepine are chemically similar to a TCA-D, and concurrent administration is not recommended.
MAO-I	Meperidine	Concurrent administration has resulted in serious toxicity and death in adult patients.
MAO-I	Dextromethorphan	Concurrent administration has resulted in excitation, hypertension, and hyperpyrexia.
MAO-I	Antipsychotic agents	Concurrent administration may prolong the sedative, hypotensive, and anticholinergic effects.
MAO-I	Sympathomimetics, CNS stimulants	Concurrent administration has reresulted in severe adverse effects including severe headache, hypertension, and hyperpyrexia. These medications should not be administered within 14 days of MAO-I therapy.
MAO-I	Antihistamines, Anticholinergics	Concurrent administration may result in increased anticholinergic or antihistamine effect. Concurrent administration is not recommended.
MAO-I	Alcohol	Increased CNS depressant effects, also several alcoholic beverages contain tyramine which may induce a hypertensive crisis.

MONITORING GUIDELINES

Baseline Assessment:

- History and physical, including height and weight of the patient.

- Orthostatic blood pressures and pulse, electrocardiogram, electrolytes, and liver function tests. Other laboratory tests as indicated.
- Describe the dietary and drug restrictions, and encourage strict compliance.
- Determine the patient's ability to follow the prescribed dietary and drug restrictions.

Time Pattern for Response: In the treatment of ADHD, Zametkin et al. (1985) reported that response was immediate and comparable to dextroamphetamine. In the chart review by Ryan et al. (1988) the time pattern in the treatment of TCA-D resistant depression was not reported.

Follow-Up Assessment:

- Height and weight according to patient status.
- Orthostatic blood pressure and pulse should routinely be obtained during dose titration and during follow-up.
- Liver function tests are indicated according to patient status.
- Monitor for adverse effects that are reported in the pediatric and adult populations.

Drug Discontinuation: Abrupt discontinuation of an MAO-I is not recommended, and has been associated with nightmares in one adolescent (Ryan et al., 1988). It is recommended that the dose of an MAO-I be tapered. The dietary and drug restrictions need to be continued for two weeks following discontinuation of an MAO-I.

SPECIAL INSTRUCTIONS FOR PARENTS/CARE GIVERS/ CHILDREN/ADOLESCENTS

- Monoamine oxidase inhibitors (MAO-I) require diligent observation of dietary and drug restrictions.
- If the child or adolescent develops any signs or symptoms of MAO-I induced hypertensive crisis the patient should be taken to a hospital emergency room immediately.

- Dietary and drug restrictions are to be observed for two weeks following MAO-I discontinuation.
- Dietary restrictions include any aged, fermented, or pickled protein including cheese, sausages, fish, meat; overripe avocados, bananas, banana peel, figs, raisins; yeast extracts; soy sauce; bean curd; ginseng; sauerkraut; fava or broad bean pods; nuts; chocolate; caffeine; all alcoholic and non-alcoholic beverages. Be careful, and remember that soups, salad dressing, and other dishes may contain one of the restricted foods. Discuss any questions that you have concerning the diet restrictions with your physician or pharmacist.
- Drugs that should not be given to patients taking an MAO-I include over-the-counter cold and flu, hay fever, and weight reduction products plus many prescription drugs. Do not take or administer any other drugs without checking with your physician or pharmacist.
- Be sure to tell all physicians, pharmacists and dentists that you are taking an MAO-I.
- There are several side effects of MAO-I therapy that include feeling tired, sleepiness, decreased appetite, insomnia, headache, urinary retention, changes in blood pressure, dizziness, palpitations, blurred vision, weakness, irritability, and aggression. Report to your physician any other side effects or unusual reactions.
- MAO-I therapy may result in drowsiness or dizziness, and patients should be careful driving a car, riding a bike, or doing other tasks that require alertness.
- Store this and all medications out of the reach of the patient and other children and adolescents.

PRODUCTS AVAILABLE

Phenelzine is available as Nardil® from Parke-Davis in orange, non-scored tablets imprinted with PD270. Each tablet contains 15 mg of phenelzine.

Tranylcypromine is available as Parnate® from SmithKline Beecham in maroon, non-scored tablets imprinted with

SKF, Parnate. Each tablet contains 10 mg of tranylcypro-mine.

COST

GENERIC NAME	TRADENAME	AWP*	AWP* per dose
Phenelzine	Nardil® 15 mg	$36.67 for 100 tables	$0.37 per tablet
Tranylcypromine	Parnate® 10 mg tablets	$41.35 for 100 tablets	$0.42 per tablet

*AWP is the average wholesale price to the pharmacist that is listed in the *1994 Redbook* (Cardinale, 1994).

SELECTIVE SEROTONIN REUPTAKE BLOCKERS

Fluoxetine hydrochloride
  Prozac® is marketed by Dista.

DSM-IV INDICATIONS

Depression (???)

Obsessive-compulsive disorder (???)

Attention-Deficit/Hyperactivity Disorder (???)

Autism (???)

Anorexia (???)

> FDA: Safety and efficacy have not been established in the pediatric population (*PDR,* 1994).
> USP: Safety and efficacy have not been established in the pediatric population (*USPDI,* 1994).

CONTRAINDICATIONS: Hypersensitivity to fluoxetine, mania or hypomania, seizures or history of seizures, multiple medications (*see* Drug Interactions), impairment of renal or hepatic function, and diabetes mellitus.

PHARMACOLOGY: Fluoxetine is an oral antidepressant chemically related to amphetamine, and is chemically distinct from the tricyclic, tetracyclic, and monoamine oxidase inhibitor antidepressants. As a selective inhibitor of serotonin uptake in the central nervous system, fluoxetine increases the activity of serotonin. Fluoxetine has minimal effect on cholinergic, histaminergic, dopaminergic, or alpha-adrenergic receptors. The major metabolite of fluoxetine is norfluoxetine, which also inhibits serotonin uptake. Fluoxetine is used in adults in the treatment of depression and obsessive compulsive disorder.

STUDIES OF FLUOXETINE EFFICACY

Depression

Simeon et al. (1990) reported a negative double-blind, placebo-controlled study of the effects of fluoxetine in the treatment of 30 adolescents with depression. The study design included a one-week trial of single-blind placebo treatment to identify and exclude placebo responders. Patients, ages 13 to 18 years, were randomly assigned to fluoxetine or placebo in the seven week trial. Fluoxetine was initiated at 20 mg per day, was increased after four days to 40 mg, and to 60 mg during the second week. Further dosage adjustments were done according to response. Patients were contacted eight to 46 months after the study ended to assess psychosocial adaptation ratings at follow-up. These ratings were obtained from patients, parents, and clinicians. Fluoxetine treatment was not statistically superior to placebo either during the trial or during the subsequent follow-up phase. There was no relationship between dose and plasma levels of fluoxetine or norfluoxetine, or between plasma levels and response to fluoxetine. The most frequently reported side effects were headache, vomiting, insomnia, rhinitis, weight loss, and tremor. This preliminary controlled trial suggests that further trials with a larger number of patients will need to be conducted to determine the effectiveness of fluoxetine in the treatment of adolescent depression.

Subsequent to the study by Simeon et al. (1990) there are two reports of open trials of fluoxetine in the treatment of major depression (Boulos et al., 1992; Jain et al., 1992). Jain et al. (1992) reviewed the charts of 31 hospitalized children or adolescents (ages nine to 18 years) treated with fluoxetine. Fluoxetine doses of 20 to 80 mg per day were administered. After 35 days of fluoxetine therapy, 54 percent of the patients were much to very much improved on the Clinical Global Impressions scale. The most common side effects were hypomanic-like symptoms, irritability, gastrointestinal upset, and insomnia. Each of the four patients that were in the depressed phase of bipolar disorder experienced hypomania. Fluoxetine was discontinued in 28 percent of the patients due to irritability, hypomanic-like symptoms, and nonresponse. None of the patients experienced sedation, weight changes, anticholinergic effects, seizures, suicidal ideation or behavior, blood pressure changes, or effects on the electrocardiogram. Concurrent medications administered included lithium, neuroleptics, and methylphenidate. The response rate in this study is comparable to placebo response rates in other studies of depression in children and adolescents. The high doses used in this study may account for the frequency of side effects. Lower doses of fluoxetine 20 mg per day are currently recommended for the treatment of depression in adults.

Boulos et al. (1992) reported 11 cases of adolescent or young adults (16 to 24 years) who were nonresponsive to tricyclic antidepressant therapy, and treated with fluoxetine and individual therapy. Of these patients 64 percent showed a therapeutic response with a 50 percent or greater reduction in symptoms on the Hamilton Depression Rating Scale. Concurrent medications included lithium, clonazepam, and valproic acid, and were administered to six of the patients. Side effects were reported as mild and consisted of tremor, dry mouth, nausea, sweating, alopecia, skin rash, and decreased appetite. One patient became manic, but none showed an increase in suicidal ideations. Fluoxetine doses ranged from 5 to 40 mg per day. The authors suggest that lower doses of fluoxetine may be effective and associated with less side effects (Boulos et al., 1992). Based on the studies above, fluoxetine is minimally effective, if at all, in the treatment of depression and is associated with a substantial incidence of side effects. More double-blind, placebo-controlled studies are indicated to determine the efficacy and adverse effect profile of fluoxetine in the treatment of depression.

Obsessive-Compulsive Disorder

Open studies suggest that fluoxetine may be effective in the treatment of children or adolescents with obsessive compulsive disorder (Como and Kurlan, 1991; Liebowitz et al., 1990; Riddle et al., 1990a). To be considered a responder, the patient had to demonstrate a 50 percent reduction in the time spent on obsessions and compulsions. These studies report a 50 percent response rate with a large percentage of fluoxetine discontinuation due to nonresponse or side effects.

Two double-blind, placebo-controlled studies of the treatment of fluoxetine in obsessive-compulsive disorder are reported (Kurlan et al., 1993; Riddle et al., 1992). The study by Kurlan et al. (1993) included 11 boys, aged ten to 18 years (mean age of 13.1 years), with Tourette's syndrome and associated obsessive compulsive symptoms. Patients were randomly assigned to placebo or fluoxetine, and six patients were allowed to maintain their current haloperidol or clonidine therapy for tics. Fluoxetine 20 mg per day was administered for two months, followed by an increase to 40 mg if the medication was tolerated. The authors reported no significant differences between treatment groups for the obsessive compulsive symptoms. Fluoxetine therapy was associated with a trend toward some improvement in tic severity, attentional abilities, and social functioning. Side effects observed included hypomanic behavior, irritability, fatigue, and agitation.

Riddle et al. (1992) reported a randomized, double-blind, crossover study of 13 children, ages eight to 15 years, treated with a 20 mg fixed dose of fluoxetine. The study design was 20 weeks long with crossover at eight weeks. No additional psychotropics were administered during the study, but seven patients continued with psychotherapy. Only six of the 13 patients finished the full 20 weeks of the study. Statistical analysis of the first eight weeks showed that patients taking fluoxetine were more improved than patients taking placebo on the Clinical Global Impressions scale, but there was no difference in the symptoms of the obsessive compulsive disorder. Side effects observed included insomnia, fatigue, increased motor activity, and nausea. Both of these double-blind studies and the open studies suggest that fluoxetine is minimally effective in the treatment of patients with obsessive compulsive symptoms. Further studies assessing the effect of dose and concurrent therapies need to be conducted.

Attention-Deficit/Hyperactivity Disorder

Barrickman et al. (1991) reported the use of fluoxetine in 19 children and adolescents with attention-deficit/hyperactivity disorder (ADHD). The patients were seven to 15 years of age with a mean of 10.9 years, and 14 of the patients had a concurrent conduct or oppositional defiant disorder. Most of the patients were treatment resistant or only partially responsive. Some of the patients had experienced adverse effects from previous medication for ADHD. The patients were administered 20 to 60 mg of fluoxetine (mean of 27 mg) per day over the six-week trial. At completion of the trial, 58 percent of the patients were rated at least moderately improved. Reported side effects include mild sedation, facial rash, feeling "spacey" and possible akathesia. The authors suggest that fluoxetine may offer an alternative in the treatment of ADHD, especially in treatment resistant cases or for patients who have side effects from other medications (Barrickman, et al.) Further double-blind, placebo-controlled studies are warranted.

Anorexia

A case report by Lyles, Sarkis, and Kemph (1990) describes the successful use of fluoxetine 20 mg/day in the treatment of a 16-year-old female for anorexia and bulimia nervosa, and major depression. Within two weeks the patient demonstrated a remarkable improvement and no longer experienced depression, irritability, impulsivity, binging or purging, distorted body image, or food craving. The patient steadily gained weight and remained symptom free at a six-month follow-up. The patient reported no side effects. This preliminary report suggests that fluoxetine may be useful in the treatment of eating disorders.

Autism

A preliminary report by Cook et al. (1992) suggests that fluoxetine may improve the functioning in patients with autism or mental retardation. This open trial included 23 subjects with autistic disorder, and 16 subjects with mental retardation. A diagnostically heterogeneous group of patients were studied. Patients were allowed to continue a variety of concomitant psychotropic medications. Fifteen of 23 patients with autism and ten of 16 patients with mental retardation were improved with fluoxetine treatment. Signs and symptoms that improved in individual patients were compulsive activity, agitation, aggressiveness, and mood. Side effects were frequent and included hyperactivity, restlessness, insomnia, elated affect, decreased appetite, increased rate of screaming, and extrapyramidal effects. This report requires replication in a more diagnostically homogeneous group of patients who are not taking concurrent medications.

DEVELOPMENTAL PHARMACOKINETICS

(Pharmacokinetic studies have not been conducted in children or adolescents.)

Absorption: Food does not affect the extent of absorption but may reduce the rate of absorption. In adults, peak plasma levels occur six to eight hours after a single dose.

Onset of action: Depending upon the condition treated, response may be seen within one to eight weeks.

Metabolism: Fluoxetine is metabolized in the liver to an active metabolite, norfluoxetine, and other metabolites.

Half-life: In adults, the elimination half-life of fluoxetine is two to three days, and seven to nine days for norfluoxetine.

Plasma levels: Plasma level studies have not been reported in the pediatric population.

DOSAGE RANGES

Fluoxetine dose finding studies have not been conducted. Doses utilized in efficacy studies range from 5 to 80 mg per day. Recently published studies have used lower doses for children, adolescents, and in the adult populations. Lower initial doses of 5 to 10 mg are suggested, followed by gradual increases in dose every one to two weeks. Due to the long half-life of fluoxetine and norfluoxetine, steady-state plasma levels may not be reached in some patients for two to three weeks.

ADVERSE EFFECTS REPORTED IN CHILDREN AND ADOLESCENTS

COMMON

In the efficacy studies described above the following adverse effects were observed: headache, nausea, vomiting, insomnia, decreased appetite, weight loss, fatigue, tremor, hypomania, hyperactivity, irritability, agitation, feeling "spacey," akathesia, restlessness, elated affect, giggling, extrapyramidal effects, dry mouth, sweating, skin rash, rhinitis, alopecia, and increased rate of screaming. The additional adverse effects of social disinhibition and a subjective sensation of excitation have been reported (Riddle, 1990/1991).

UNCOMMON

Due to the lack of extended treatment studies, there is a lack of information in this area. Practitioners are encouraged to monitor for the adverse effects that have been reported for adults until further information is available (*see also* Adverse Reactions/Case Reports).

ALLERGIC REACTION: Symptoms of an allergic reaction include skin rash; hives; tingling or burning of the fingers, hands, or arms; chills or fever; swollen glands; joint or muscle pain; swelling of the feet or lower legs; or trouble in breathing.

TOXICITY: Agitation, restlessness, hypomania, severe nausea or vomiting, and seizures are signs and symptoms of fluoxetine toxicity (*see* Adverse Reactions/Case Reports).

ADVERSE REACTIONS/CASE REPORTS

Fluoxetine-Induced Mania

Mania or hypomania associated with fluoxetine therapy has been reported in a total of five separate case reports involving one ten-year-old child, and eight adolescents aged 13 to 16 years (Achamallah and Decker, 1991; Jafri, 1991; Jerome, 1991; Rosenberg, Johnson, and Sahl, 1992; Venkataraman, Naylor, and King, 1992). Symptoms of mania usually start within one week after initiation of fluoxetine therapy and do not appear to be related to dose. Signs and symptoms include the usual manifestations of mania: pressured speech, increased motor activity, decreased need for sleep, hypersexuality, impulsiveness, aggressiveness, giggling, and laughing. Predisposing factors to the development of fluoxetine-induced mania include a family history of bipolar disorder or other affective illnesses, or concurrent symptoms of attention-deficit/hyperactivity disorder or psychosis (Venkataraman, Naylor, and King, 1992). The mania resolved for each patient within two weeks of discontinuation of fluoxetine. An interesting observation is that in the case report by Achamallah and Decker (1991) the patient developed mania while taking an antipsychotic, thiothixene 40 mg per day. There is also a single case report of a seven-year-old child who developed mania while taking sertraline (Ghaziuddin, 1994). Sertraline is also a selective serotonin reuptake inhibitor. As in adults, the use of a selective serotonin reuptake inhibitor may be associated with the onset of manic-like symptoms.

Fluoxetine Overdose

Riddle et al. (1989) reported the case of a 13-year-old boy who intentionally ingested an estimated 1.88 grams of fluoxetine in a suicide attempt. The patient denied taking any other medications. The patient was admitted to the emergency room 45 to 75 minutes after the overdose. After 30 ml of ipecac was administered, 500 ml of vomitus was produced that contained no signs of capsules. The patient was alert and responsive with normal vital signs and neurological examination. Approximately three hours after the ingestion, the patient had a generalized tonic-clonic seizure that lasted two to three minutes. The patient was treated with intravenous diazepam, phenytoin, and oral-activated charcoal. This was followed in one hour by 150 ml of magnesium citrate and intravenous sodium bicarbonate 50 mEq. The electrocardiogram at this time revealed depressed ST segments but was otherwise normal. The fluoxetine level obtained 90 minutes after the ingestion was 427.8 ng/ml and the norfluoxetine (major active metabolite of fluoxetine) level was 210.9 ng/ml. A repeat serum level 15 hours after the ingestion showed a fluoxetine level of 1142 ng/ml and a norfluoxetine level of 322 ng/ml. The patient at this time complained of blurred vision, tiredness, frontal headache, and dizziness. A third blood sample 66 hours after ingestion showed a fluoxetine level of 449.5 ng/ml and a norfluoxetine level of 247 ng/ml. The authors report that all of the signs and symptoms remitted spontaneously, and the patient was transferred to a psychiatric facility for further care (Riddle et al., 1989).

Fluoxetine and Galactorrhea with Hyperprolactinemia

Iancu et al. (1992) reported a 17-year-old female who was treated with fluoxetine for anorexia and bulimia nervosa, depression, and suicidal behavior. The patient was treated with 60 mg of fluoxetine a day with a starting dose of 20 mg per day. Within two weeks she developed galactorrhea and hyperprolactinemia of 50 ng/ml (prolactin reference range is 0 to 18 ng/ml). The dose of fluoxetine was reduced to 40 mg per day, and the galactorrhea stopped, and the prolactin levels returned to normal (Iancu et al., 1992) . The finding of hyperprolactinemia has also been reported in adults.

Fluoxetine and Self-Injurious Behavior

King et al. (1991) reported six patients receiving fluoxetine that developed or experienced an exacerbation in self-injurious behavior or ideation. The patients received fluoxetine for obsessive compulsive disorder but had comorbid diagnoses of Tourette's syndrome, oppositional disorder, social and separation anxiety, and probable dysthymic disorder. Three of the patients had a history of prior suicidal ideation, one of whom also had a history of self-injurious behavior. The onset of the symptoms occurred within one month for three patients, within two months for one patient, and after six months or more of fluoxetine therapy for two patients. The authors suggest three possible explanations for the emergence of the suicidal ideation and self-destructive behavior in these children or adolescents. First, the self-destructive behavior is coincidentally related to fluoxetine therapy. Second, fluoxetine may have induced the agitation, disorganization, or mood changes that resulted in these symptoms. Third, fluoxetine may have had a specific effect on the regulation of aggression directed either outward or toward the self. The authors acknowledge that like all psychotropics, the effects of fluoxetine are complex and variable, and practitioners need to carefully monitor for potentially serious adverse effects (King et al., 1991).

Fluoxetine and Psychosis

Hersh, Sokol, and Pfeffer (1991) reported the case of an 11-year-old girl who was treated for major depression and suicidal ideation. The child had a history of previous head trauma and her electroencephalogram (EEG) was abnormal with intermittent sharp waves and bursts of theta slowing bilaterally, synchronously, and asynchronously, but there were no known seizures. The patient was treated with fluoxetine with varying doses of 10 to 20 mg per day. After 35 days of treatment the patient's mood became less depressed, her affect brightened, and her sleep patterns normalized. The dose of fluoxetine was subsequently lowered to 20 mg every other day. After eight days of alternate day therapy the patient became delusional and desolate. Fluoxetine was discontinued, and the delusional material remitted within 24 hours. The authors suggest that the history of head trauma and the abnormal EEG may have contributed to this child's susceptibility to develop psychosis associated with fluoxetine administration (Hersh, Sokol, and Pfeffer, 1991).

Fluoxetine and Tics

Eisenhauer and Jermain (1993) reported a case of a 12-year-old male who was treated with fluoxetine 20 mg per day for major depression without psychotic features. No adverse effects were noted for eight months. At this point the patient began to have numerous tics consisting of eye-blinking, shoulder hunching, and in and out movements of the abdomen. The tics gradually worsened, and the fluoxetine was discontinued. The tics completely abated six months later. Although the authors refer to the movements as tics, they also described the movements in terms of abnormal involuntary movements. The authors suggest that the effects of fluoxetine on serotonin, an inhibitory neurotransmitter, may affect dopaminergic neurons. The authors describe several case reports of adults who developed extrapyramidal reactions while taking fluoxetine and suggest that practitioners monitor for potentially severe extrapyramidal adverse reactions in all patients taking fluoxetine.

DRUG INTERACTIONS

DRUG	DRUGS	EFFECT
Fluoxetine	Monoamine oxidase inhibitors	Serotonin syndrome, a potentially lethal hyperserotonergic state, may result in the combination of an MAO-I and fluoxetine. Concurrent use is contraindicated. MAO-I therapy should be discontinued two weeks before initiation of fluoxetine. Fluoxetine therapy should be discontinued for five weeks before initiation of MAO-I therapy.
Fluoxetine	Lithium	Increased lithium levels may occur resulting in lithium toxicity. Monitoring of lithium serum levels is indicated.
Fluoxetine	Tricyclic antidepressants, Clomipramine, Trazodone, Maprotiline	Increased plasma levels of the tricyclic antidepressants may occur, and monitoring of tricyclic antidepressant plasma levels is indicated (March, Moon, and Johnston, 1990; DeMaso and Hunter, 1990). Dosage reductions up to 50 percent may be required.
Fluoxetine	Carbamazepine, Phenytoin	An increase in serum carbamazepine levels may occur, and monitoring of the carbamazepine serum level is indicated.
Fluoxetine	Neuroleptics	Increased adverse effects including agitation, irritability, aggression, and extrapyramidal effects have been reported when neuroleptics and fluoxetine are used concurrently (Eisenhauer and Jermain, 1993; Matthews et al., 1991).

Fluoxetine	Dextromethorphan	Hallucinations have occurred during concurrent use.
Fluoxetine	Sympathomimetics, Phenylpropanolamine	Concurrent use of fluoxetine and diets aids or central nervous system stimulants may result in increased heart rate, dizziness, diarrhea, and increased weight loss (Walter, 1992).
Fluoxetine	Tryptophan	Concurrent administration may result in agitation, restlessness, and gastrointestinal problems.
Fluoxetine	Alcohol, other CNS depressants	Fluoxetine may potentiate central nervous system depression if used concurrently.
Fluoxetine	Digoxin, Warfarin	Fluoxetine is highly protein bound and may displace other plasma protein bound drugs. Monitoring the effects of digoxin and warfarin are suggested.

MONITORING GUIDELINES

Baseline Assessment:

- History and physical, including weight of the patient.
- Routine laboratory profile as indicated by patient status.

Time Pattern for Response:

- Depending upon the disorder treated responses have occurred within one to eight weeks.

Follow-Up Assessment:

- Patients should be monitored for response and for adverse effects. There are no routine laboratory tests currently indicated during fluoxetine therapy.
- Many of the common adverse effects (insomnia, agitation, restlessness, and social disinhibition) may respond to dosage (Riddle, 1990/1991).

Drug Discontinuation:

- Like all psychotropic medications, the dose of fluoxetine should be reduced and then discontinued. The long half-life of fluoxetine results in a gradual reduction in plasma levels.

SPECIAL INSTRUCTIONS FOR PARENTS/CARE GIVERS/CHILDREN/ADOLESCENTS

- Side effects of fluoxetine that may occur are nausea, weight loss or gain, anxiety or nervousness, insomnia, excessive sweating, and headaches. Report these side effects to your physician if they continue or are bothersome to the patient.
- Fluoxetine may cause drowsiness during the first few weeks of therapy. If this happens, the patient should not participate in activities that require alertness, such a riding a bike or driving a car.
- Some persons may become restless or agitated with increased activity, rapid speech, or a feeling of being "speeded up" while taking fluoxetine. Report to your physician as soon as possible if any of these side effects occur.
- If the patient develops a skin rash or hives, stop the fluoxetine and check with the physician as soon as possible.
- Be sure to let all physicians, pharmacists, and other health care practitioners know that you are taking fluoxetine.
- Be sure to contact your doctor if you feel you are not getting better or if you develop any unusual reactions to fluoxetine.
- Do not take any other medications while taking fluoxetine without checking with your physician or pharmacist.
- Store this medication and all medications away from the patient and other children and adolescents.

PRODUCTS AVAILABLE

Fluoxetine hydrochloride is available as Prozac® from Dista Pharmaceutical.

Prozac® 10 mg is marketed in green and gray capsules. Prozac® 20 mg is marketed in 20 mg green and off-white capsules. Prozac® syrup contains 20 mg of fluoxetine in 5 ml and is mint flavored.

COST

GENERIC NAME	TRADENAME	AWP*	AWP* per dose
Fluoxetine	Prozac® 10 mg	$203.29 for 100 capsules	$2.04 per capsule
	Prozac® 20 mg	$208.52 for 100 capsules	$2.09 per capsule
	Prozac® syrup 20 mg per 5 ml	$389.79 for 500 ml	$3.86 per 5 ml

* AWP is the average wholesale price to the pharmacist that is listed in the *1994 Redbook* (Cardinale, 1994).

TRAZODONE

Trazodone hydrochloride

Desyrel® is marketed by Mead Johnson Pharmaceuticals. Trazodone is also available in generic form.

DSM-IV INDICATIONS

Conduct/Oppositional Defiant Disorder, aggression (???)

FDA: Safety and efficacy have not been established in pediatric populations (*PDR,* 1994).

USP: Appropriate studies on the relationship of age to the effects of trazodone have not been performed in the pediatric population (*USPDI,* 1994).

CONTRAINDICATIONS: Hypersensitivity to trazodone, previous occurrence of priapism, prolonged penile erections during trazodone therapy, pregnancy, cardiovascular disorders, hepatic, or renal impairment.

PHARMACOLOGY: Trazodone hydrochloride is a triazolopyridine antidepressant that selectively inhibits the reuptake of serotonin and potentiates the activity of serotonin. Animal studies indicate that trazodone acts as a serotonin agonist at high doses (6 to 8 mg/kg) while at low doses (0.05 to 1.0 mg/kg) it acts as an antagonist. Trazodone also causes beta-receptor subsensitivity or decreases the number of beta-adrenergic binding sites. Trazodone is not a monoamine oxidase inhibitor or a tricyclic antidepressant and does not stimulate the central nervous system. Trazodone has significant sedative, anxiolytic, and analgesic effects.

STUDIES OF TRAZODONE EFFICACY

Aggression

Three clinical reports have described the effects of trazodone in the treatment of aggression (Fras, 1987; Ghaziuddin and Alessi,

1992; Zubieta and Alessi, 1992). Fras (1987) described a 15-year-old boy with oppositional defiant disorder and a dysphoric mood who was treated with 200 mg of trazodone daily. The patient responded with reduced levels of aggression that was maintained over eight months of follow-up. No side effects were reported (Fras, 1987). Ghaziuddin and Alessi (1992) reported on the effects of trazodone in three prepubertal children whose primary diagnoses were disruptive disorders and aggression. In each case, the aggression responded to trazodone 3 to 3.5 mg/kg/day. There was no reported effect of trazodone on the symptoms of attention-deficit/hyperactivity disorder in one patient. In each case, the medication was discontinued for various reasons, e.g., noncompliance, and aggression returned within a few days. The symptoms of aggression were decreased upon the reinitiation of trazodone. Side effects did not require discontinuation of trazodone in any of the patients. One patient showed mild sedation, and one patient experienced two spontaneous penile erections. For this patient, the dose of trazodone was reduced from 100 mg per day to 75 mg per day with no further reported problems. No cardiovascular side effects or electrocardiogram abnormalities were reported. The authors suggest that trazodone had an antiaggression effect for these children and not an antidepressant effect. Trazodone in the treatment of child and adolescent depression has not been reported.

Zubieta and Alessi (1992) reported an open trial of trazodone in the treatment of severe behavioral disturbances in 22 hospitalized children (aged five to 12 years) who were unresponsive to other treatments. Trazodone was initiated at 50 mg at night and increased to the maximal tolerated dose by the end of the first week of therapy. Thirteen patients were found to benefit from trazodone therapy. Aggressive, impulsive behaviors were the symptoms that improved the most with trazodone therapy. Improvement was not associated with sedative effects. Three of the nonresponders, actually became worse on trazodone therapy with increased irritability, temper tantrums, and self-injurious behavior. Orthostatic hypotension was the most frequently reported adverse effect requiring discontinuation in one patient. Tolerance to the orthostatic effect was noted within two to three days after achieving maximal doses. Drowsiness, increased nervousness, increased fatigue, and nocturnal enuresis were also reported. One child reported painful erections without priapism that required discontinuation of trazodone. The authors acknowledge that further studies are required to determine the role of trazodone in the treatment of disruptive behavioral disorders (Zubieta and Alessi, 1992).

DEVELOPMENTAL PHARMACOKINETICS

Absorption: Trazodone is well absorbed after oral administration in adults. In adults, peak plasma levels occur in one hour when administered on an empty stomach and in two hours when taken with food.

Onset of action: The onset of antiaggressive effects were noted within one week (Ghaziuddin and Alessi, 1992).

Half-life: The half-life of trazodone in adults is biphasic. The initial half-life is three to six hours followed by a five- to nine-hour half-life. The half-life is not reported in children.

Plasma levels: Plasma levels have not been correlated to therapeutic response.

DOSAGE RANGE

Aggression: In the two open trials of trazodone in the treatment of aggression, doses were initiated at 1.0 mg/kg/day. Doses were increased every three to four days, according to response and adverse effects. Maximal doses administered ranged from 3.0 to 6.0 mg/kg/day. Due to the presumed short half-life of trazodone in the pediatric population (this has not been evaluated), trazodone was administered in three divided daily doses (Zubieta and Alessi, 1992). It is recommended to administer trazodone with food to decrease the rate of absorption and the maximum serum concentrations. Slower absorption may decrease the nausea or dizziness associated with peak serum concentrations of trazodone.

ADVERSE EFFECTS REPORTED IN CHILDREN AND ADOLESCENTS

COMMON

Orthostatic hypotension, sedation, increased nervousness, increased fatigue, nocturnal enuresis, painful penile erections, and worsening of behavior have been reported in two preliminary reports of trazodone (Ghaziuddin and Alessi, 1992; Zubieta and Alessi, 1992).

LESS COMMON

Due to the lack of studies, there is a lack of information in this area. Until further information is available, practitioners are encouraged to monitor for the adverse effects that have been reported in adults. Trazodone, a drug with alpha-blocking activity, is associated with priapism. Priapism is defined as a pathologically prolonged painful erection of the penis involving the corpora cavernosa, while the corpus spongiosum and glans penis remain flaccid. Several drugs with alpha-blocking activity are associated with priapism. The incidence of trazodone-induced priapism in adults is 1 in 1,000 or less. From the studies described above which included a total of 26 patients, two patients developed painful or spontaneous penile erections. Based on these preliminary reports the incidence of this adverse effect may be higher in the pediatric population. Patients should be informed of this effect and warned to discontinue the medication and contact their physician if prolonged erections occur. Patients need to be aware that prolonged erections are not a favorable side effect and should be encouraged to immediately report an occurrence. Prior to the onset of priapism, 50 percent of patients report a history of prolonged erections. In adults, priapism is associated with doses of 150 mg or less and frequently occurs during the first 28 days of therapy. Priapism may require surgical intervention and may result in urinary retention, impairment of erec-

tile function or impotence (Thompson, Ware, and Blashfield, 1990).

ALLERGIC REACTION: In adult patients, trazodone therapy has resulted in an allergic skin reaction with pruritis
and urticaria.

TOXICITY: Signs and symptoms of toxicity that have been
reported in adults include drowsiness, loss of muscle
coordination, nausea, and vomiting.

DRUG INTERACTIONS

DRUG	DRUGS	EFFECT
Trazodone	Alcohol, barbiturates, CNS depressants, Antidepressants, Antipsychotics	Trazodone may enhance the sedative and acticholinergic effects of these drugs.
Trazodone	Digoxin	Serum levels of digoxin have been increased with trazodone administration. Monitoring of digoxin serum levels is indicated.
Trazodone	Phenytoin	Phenytoin serum levels have been increased with trazodone administration. Monitoring of phenytoin serum levels is indicated.
Trazodone	Warfarin	Trazodone administration may increase effects of warfarin.
Trazodone	Antihistamines, Anticholinergics	Concurrent administration may result in increased anticholinergic or antihistamine effect. Concurrent administration is not recommended.
Trazodone	Monoamine oxidase	Concurrent administration has not been evaluated, but caution is indicated.

MONITORING GUIDELINES

Baseline Assessment:

- History and physical, including weight and height of the patient.
- Orthostatic blood pressure and pulse, electrocardiogram, white blood cell count with differential, and liver function tests. Other laboratory tests as indicated.

Time Pattern for Response:

- Preliminary reports indicate the effects of trazodone on aggression are evident within one week of therapy (Ghaziuddin and Alessi, 1992).

Follow-Up Assessment:

- Orthostatic blood pressure and pulse should routinely be obtained during dose titration and during follow-up.
- In adults, low white blood cell and neutrophil counts have been noted, but were not considered to be clinically significant. Trazodone therapy should be discontinued if the white blood cell or neutrophil counts fall below normal. White blood cell counts with differentials are indicated if a patient develops a fever, sore throat, or other signs of infection. The implications of this finding for children or adolescents is unknown.
- Other laboratory tests and procedures as patient status indicates.

Drug Discontinuation:

- Abrupt discontinuation is not recommended. Tapering of the dose according to response or adverse effects is recommended.

SPECIAL INSTRUCTIONS FOR PARENTS/CARE GIVERS/ CHILDREN/ADOLESCENTS

- Trazodone should be taken with food, which will help decrease stomach upset and dizziness.
- Trazodone therapy may result in drowsiness or dizziness, and patients should be careful driving a car, riding a bike or doing other tasks that require alertness.
- Trazodone therapy in male patients has been rarely associated with prolonged, inappropriate, and painful penile erections. If this happens, immediately discontinue trazodone therapy and contact the physician.
- Patients taking trazodone should avoid taking alcohol or other depressant drugs.
- Store this medication and all medications away from the patient and other children and adolescents.

PRODUCTS AVAILABLE

Trazodone hydrochloride is available as Desyrel® from Mead Johnson and as a generic product. Desyrel® is marketed in a 50 mg, round, orange, scored tablet imprinted with MG 775 Desyrel; a 100 mg, round, white, scored tablet imprinted with MG 776 Desyrel; a 150 mg, orange, triple scored, tablet imprinted with MJ 778 50; and a 300 mg, yellow, triple scored tablet imprinted with MJ 796 100 dosage forms. Desyrel® 150 mg tablets may be divided to yield doses of 50, 75, or 100 mg. Desyrel® 300 mg tablets may be divided to yield three doses of 100 mg, two doses of 150 mg, or one dose of 200 mg.

Trazodone is available in generic form as 50 mg, 100 mg, and 150 mg tablets.

COST

GENERIC NAME	TRADENAME	AWP*	AWP* per dose
Trazodone 50 mg		$8.93 for 100 tablets	$0.09 per tablet
Trazodone 100 mg		$12.75 for 100 tablets	$0.13 per tablet
Trazodone 150 mg		$56.93 for 100 tablets	$0.57 per tablet
	Desyrel® 50 mg	$118.44 for 100 tablets	$1.19 per tablet
	Desyrel® 100 mg	$206.99 for 100 tablets	$2.07 per tablet
	Desyrel® 150 mg	$178.33 for 100 tablets	$1.79 per tablet
	Desyrel® 300 mg	$317.39 for 100 tablets	$3.18 per tablet

*AWP is the average wholesale price to the pharmacist that is listed in the *1994 Redbook* (Cardinale, 1994).

REFERENCES

Tricyclic Antidepressants

Abramowicz, M (ed). Sudden death in children treated with a tricyclic antidepressant. *Med Lett Drugs Ther,* 1990;32:53.

Akiskal, HS, Mallya, G. Criteria for the "soft" bipolar spectrum: Treatment implications. *Psychopharmacol Bull,* 1987;23:68-73.

Alarcon, RD, Johnson, BR, Lucas, JP. Paranoid and aggressive behavior in two obsessive-compulsive adolescents treated with clomipramine. *J Amer Acad Child Adolesc Psychiatry,* 1991;30:999-1002.

Ambrosini, PJ, Bianchi, MD, Rabinovich, H, Elia, J. Antidepressant treatments in children and adolescents. I. Affective disorder. *J Amer Acad Child Adolesc Psychiatry,* 1993;32:1-6.

Ambrosini, PJ, Bianchi, MD, Rabinovich, H, Elia, J. The safety of desipramine (letter). *J Amer Acad Child Adolesc Psychiatry,* 1994;33:590.

Baldessarini, RJ, Teicher, MH, Cassidy, JW, Stein, MH. Anticonvulsant cotreatment may increase toxic metabolites of antidepressants and other psychotropic drugs. *J Clin Psychopharmacol,* 1988;8:381-382.

Bartels, MG, Varley, CK, Mitchell, J, Stamm, SJ. Pediatric cardiovascular effects of imipramine and desipramine. *J Amer Acad Child Adolesc Psychiatry,* 1991;30:100-103.

Berney, T, Kolvin, I, Bhate, SR, Garside, RF, Jeans, J, Scarth, L. School phobia: A therapeutic trial with clomipramine and short-term outcome. *Brit J Psych,* 1981;138:110-118.

Bernstein, GA, Garfinkel, BD, Borchardt, CM. Comparative studies of pharmacotherapy for school refusal. *J Amer Acad Child Adolesc Psychiatry,* 1990;29:773-781.

Biederman, J. Pharmacological treatment of adolescents with affective disorders and attention deficit disorder. *Psychopharmacol Bull,* 1988a;24:81-87.

Biederman, J, Gastfriend, DR, Jellinek, MS. Desipramine in the treatment of children with attention deficit disorder. *J Clin Psychopharmacol*, 1986;6: 359-363.

Biederman, J, Gonzalez, E, Bronstein, B, DeMonaco, H, Wright, V. Desipramine and cutaneous reactions in pediatric outpatients. *J Clin Psych*, 1988b;49: 178-183.

Biederman, J, Baldessarini, RJ, Wright, V, Knee, D, Harmatz, JS. A double-blind placebo controlled study of desipramine in the treatment of ADD: I. Efficacy. *J Amer Acad Child Adolesc Psychiatry*, 1989a;28:777-784.

Biederman, J, Baldessarini, RJ, Wright, V, Keenan, K, Faraone, S. A double-blind placebo controlled study of desipramine in the treatment of ADD. III. Lack of impact of comorbidity and family history factors on clinical response. *J Amer Acad Child Adolesc Psychiatry*, 1993a;32:199-204.

Biederman, J, Baldessarini, RJ, Wright, V, Knee, D, Harmatz, JS, Goldblatt, A. A double-blind placebo controlled study of desipramine in the treatment of ADD: II. Serum drug levels and cardiovascular findings. *J Amer Acad Child Adolesc Psychiatry*, 1989b;28:903-911.

Biederman, J, Baldessarini, RJ, Goldblatt, A, Lapey, KA, Doyle, A, Hesslein, PS. A naturalistic study of 24-hour electrocardiographic recordings and echocardiographic findings in children and adolescents treated with desipramine. *J Amer Acad Child Adolesc Psychiatry*, 1993b;32:805-813.

Boulos, C, Kutcher, S, Marton, P, Simeon, J, Ferguson, B, Roberts, N. Response to desipramine treatment in adolescent major depression. *Psychopharm Bull*, 1991;27:59-65.

Brown, CS, Wells, BG, Cold, JA, Froemming, JH, Self, TH, Jabbour, JT. Possible influence of carbamazepine on plasma imipramine concentrations in children with attention deficit hyperactivity disorder. *J Clin Psychopharmacol*, 1990; 10:359-362.

Cardinale, VA (ed). *1994 Drug Topics Redbook*, Medical Economics Company, Inc., 1994; 96, 103, 111, 159, 183, 184, 243, 308, 388.

Cox, WH. An indication for use of imipramine in attention deficit disorder. *Am J Psych*, 1982;139:1059-1060.

Cruz, R. Clomipramine side effects. *J Amer Acad Child Adolesc Psychiatry*, 1992;31:1168-1169.

De la Fuente, JM. Carbamazepine-induced low plasma levels of tricyclic antidepressants. *J Clin Psychopharm*, 1992;12:67-68.

DeVeaugh-Geiss, J, Moroz, G, Biederman, J, Cantwell, DG, Fontaine, R, Greist, JH, Reichler, R, Katz, R, Landau, P. Clomipramine hydrochloride in childhood and adolescent obsessive-compulsive disorder: A multicenter trial. *J Amer Acad Child Adolesc Psychiatry*, 1992;31:45-49.

Diamond, JM. TCA toxicity. *J Amer Acad Child Adolesc Psychiatry*, 1993;32: 1307-1308.

Donnelly, M, Zametkin, AJ, Rapoport, JL, Ismond, DR, Weingartner, H, Lane, E, Oliver, J, Linnoila, M, Potter, WZ. Treatment of childhood hyperactivity with desipramine: Plasma drug concentration, cardiovascular effects, plasma and urinary catecholamine levels, and clinical response. *Clin Pharmacol Ther,* 1986;39:72-81.

Fernandez De Gatta, MM, Galindo, P, Gutierrez, J, Tamayo, M, Garcia, MJ, Dominguez-Gill, A. The influence of clinical and pharmacological factors on enuresis treatment with imipramine. *Br J Clin Pharmac,* 1990;30:693-698.

Fetner, HH, Geller, B. Lithium and tricyclic antidepressants. *Psych Clinics North Amer,* 1992;15:223-241.

Flament, MF, Rapoport, JL, Berg, CJ, Flament, MF, Rapoport, JL, Berg, CJ, Sceery, W, Kilts, C, Mellstrom, B, Linnoila, M. Clomipramine treatment of childhood obsessive-compulsive disorder: A double-blind controlled study. *Arch Gen Psych,* 1985;42:977-983.

Fletcher, SE, Case, CL, Sallee, FR, Hand, LD, Gillette, PC. Prospective study of the electrocardiographic effects of imipramine in children. *J Ped,* 1993;122: 652-654.

Forsythe, WI, Redmond, A. Enuresis and spontaneous cure rate: Study of 1129 enuretics. *Arch Dis Child,* 1974;49:259-263.

Fournier, JP, Garfinkel, BD, Bond, A, Beauchesne, H, Shapiro, SK. Pharmacological and behavioral management of enuresis. *J Amer Acad Child Adolesc Psychiatry,* 1987;26:849-853.

Friman, PC, Warzak, WJ. Nocturnal enuresis: A prevalent, persistent, yet curable parasomnia. *Pediatrician,* 1990;17:38-45.

Fritz, GK, Rockney, RM, Yeung, AS. Plasma levels and efficacy of imipramine treatment for enuresis. *J Amer Acad Child Adolesc Psychiatry,* 1994;33:60-64.

Furlanut, M, Montanari, G, Benetello, P, Bonin, P, Schiaulini, P, Pellegrino, PA. Steady-state serum concentrations of imipramine, its main metabolites and clinical response in primary enuresis. *Pharmacol Res,* 1989;21:561-566.

Gadow, KD. Pediatric Psychopharmacotherapy: A review of recent research. *J Child Psychol Psychiat,* 1992;33:153-195.

Garfinkel, BD, Wender, PH, Sloman, L, O'Neill, I. Tricyclic antidepressant and methylphenidate treatment of attention deficit disorder in children. *J Amer Acad Child Psychiatry,* 1983;22:343-348.

Gastfriend, DR, Biederman, J, Jellinek, MS. Desipramine in the treatment of adolescents with attention deficit disorder. *Am J Psych,* 1984;141:906-908.

Geller, B, Fox, LW, Fletcher, M. Effect of tricyclic antidepressants on switching to mania and on the onset of bipolarity in depressed 6 to 12 year olds. *J Amer Acad Child Adolesc Psychiatry,* 1993;32:43-50.

Geller, B, Cooper, TB, Chestnut, E, Abel, AS, Anker, JA. Nortriptyline pharmacokinetic parameters in depressed children and adolescents: Preliminary data. *J Clin Psychopharmacol,* 1984;4:265-269.

Geller, B, Cooper, TB, McCombs, HG, Graham, D, Wells, J. Double-blind, placebo-controlled study of nortriptyline in depressed children using a "fixed plasma level" design. *Psychopharmacol Bull,* 1989;25:101-108.

Geller, B, Cooper, TB, Graham, DL, Marsteller, FA, Bryant, DM. Double-blind, placebo-controlled study of nortriptyline in depressed adolescents using a "fixed plasma level" design. *Psychopharmacol Bull,* 1990;26:85-90.

Geller, B, Cooper, TB, Graham, DL, Fetner, HH, Marsteller, FA, Wells, JM. Pharmacokinetically designed double-blind placebo-controlled study of nortriptyline in 6 to 12 year olds with major depressive disorder. *J Amer Acad Child Adolesc Psychiatry,* 1992;31:34-44.

Ghadirian, AM, Kusalic, M. Rapid cycling following antidepressant in an adolescent. *Biol Psych,* 1990;27:1183-1184.

Gillette, DW, Tannery, LP. Beta blocker inhibits tricyclic metabolism. *J Amer Acad Child Adolesc Psychiatry,* 1994;33:223-224.

Grob, CS, Coyle, JT. Suspected adverse methylphenidate-imipramine interactions in children. *Dev Behav Pediatr,* 1986;7:265-267.

Jensen, PS, Ryan, ND, Prien, R. Psychopharmacology of child and adolescent major depression: Present status and future direction. *J Child Adolesc Psychopharmacol,* 1992;2:31-44.

Kanner, AM, Klein, RG, Rubinstein, B, Mascia, A. Use of imipramine in children with intractable asthma and psychiatric disorders: A warning. *Psychother Psychosom,* 1989;51:203-209.

Kashani, JH, Shekim, WO, Reid, JC. Amitriptyline in children with major depressive disorder: A double-blind crossover pilot study. *J Amer Acad Child Psychiatry,* 1984;23:348-351.

Klein, RG, Klein, DF. Controlled imipramine treatment of school phobia. *Arch Gen Psych,* 1971;25:204-207.

Klein, RG, Koplewicz, HS, Kanner, A. Imipramine treatment of children with separation anxiety disorder. *J Amer Acad Child Adolesc Psychiatry,* 1992;31:21-28.

Kramer, AD, Feiguine, RJ. Clinical effects of amitriptyline in adolescent depression. *J Amer Acad Child Psych,* 1981;20:636-644.

Kuekes, ED, Wigg, C, Bryant, S, Meyer, WJ. Hypertension is a risk in adolescents treated with imipramine. *J Child Adolesc Psychopharmacol,* 1992;2:241-248.

Kutcher, S, Boulos, C, Ward, B, Marton P, Simeon, S, Ferguson, B, Szalai, J, Katic, M, Roberts, N, DuBois, C, Reed, K. Response to desipramine treatment in adolescent depression: A fixed-dose, placebo-controlled trial. *J Amer Acad Child Adolesc Psychiatry,* 1994;33:686-694.

Law, W, Petti, TA, Kazdin, AE. Withdrawal symptoms after graduated cessation of imipramine in children. *Am J Psych,* 1981;138:647-650.

Leonard, HL, Swedo, SE, Rapoport, JL, Koby, EV, Lenane, MC, Cheslow, DL, Hamburger, SD. Treatment of obsessive-compulsive disorder with clomipramine and desipramine in children and adolescents: A double-blind crossover comparison. *Arch Gen Psych,* 1989;46:1088-1092.

Leonard, HL, Swedo, SE, Lenane, MC, Rettew, DC, Cheslow, DL, Hamburger, SD, Rapoport, JL. A double-blind desipramine substitution during long-term clomipramine treatment in children and adolescents with obsessive-compulsive disorder. *Arch Gen Psych,* 1991;48:922-927.

Mosholder, A, Wooldridge, JW, Bates, C. Safety of desipramine (letter). *J Amer Acad Child Adolesc Psychiatry,* 1989;28:964.

Olig, RM, Staton, RD, Beatty, WW, Wilson, H, Biberdorf, RI, Hoag, SG. Antidepressant treatment of children: Clinical relapse is unrelated to tricyclic plasma concentrations. *Perceptual Motor Skill,* 1985;60:879-889.

Parraga, HC, Cochran, MK. Emergence of motor and vocal tics during imipramine administration in two children. *J Child Adolesc Psychopharmacol,* 1992;2:227-234.

Pataki, CS, Carlson, GA, Kelly, KL, Rapport, MD, Biancaniello, TM. Side effects of methylphenidate and desipramine alone and in combination in children. *J Amer Acad Child Adolesc Psychiatry,* 1993;32:1065-1072.

Petti, TA, Law, W. Imipramine treatment of depressed children: A double-blind pilot study. *J Clin Psychopharmacol,* 1982;2:107-110.

Physician's Desk Reference. Oradell, NJ. Medical Economic Data, 1994.

Pliszka, SR. Tricyclic antidepressants in the treatment of children with attention deficit disorder. *J Amer Acad Child Adolesc Psychiatry,* 1987;26:127132.

Preskorn, SH. Pharmacokinetics of antidepressants: Why and how they are relevant to treatment. *J Clin Psych,* 1993;54:14-34.

Preskorn, SH, Weller, EB, Weller, RA. Depression in children: Relationship between plasma levels and response. *J Clin Psychiatry,* 1982;43:450-453.

Preskorn, SH, Weller, EB, Weller, RA, Glotzbach, E. Plasma levels of imipramine and adverse effects in children. *Am J Psych,* 1983;140:1332-1335.

Preskorn, SH, Weller, EB, Hughes, CW, Weller, RA. Relationship of plasma imipramine levels to CNS toxicity in children. *Am J Psych,* 1988;145:897.

Preskorn, SH, Bupp, SJ, Weller, EB, Weller, RA. Plasma levels of imipramine and metabolites in 68 hospitalized children. *J Amer Acad Child Adolesc Psychiatry,* 1989;28:373-375.

Puig-Antich, J, Perel, JM, Lupatkin, W, Chambers, WJ, Tabrizi, MA, King, J, Goetz, R, Davies M, Stiller, RL. Imipramine in prepubertal major depressive disorders. *Arch Gen Psych,* 1987;44:81-89.

Quinn, PO, Rapoport, JL. One-year follow-up of hyperactive boys treated with imipramine or methylphenidate. *Am J Psych,* 1975;132:241-245.

Rapoport, JL, Zametkin, A, Donnelly, M, Ismond, D. New drugs trials in attention deficit disorder. *Psychopharmacol Bull,* 1985;21:232-236.

Rapoport, JL, Quinn, PO, Bradbard, G, Riddle, D, Brooks, E. Imipramine and methylphenidate treatments of hyperactive boys. *Arch Gen Psych,* 1974;30:789-793.

Rapoport, JL, Mikkelsen, EJ, Zavadil, A, Nee, L, Gruenau C, Mendelson, W, Gillin, C. Childhood enuresis II. Psychopathology, tricyclic concentration in plasma, and antienuretic effect. *Arch Gen Psychiatry,* 1980;37:1146-1152.

Riddle, MA, Geller, B, Ryan, N. Another sudden death in a child treated with desipramine. *J Amer Acad Child Adolesc Psychiatry,* 1993;32:792-797.

Riddle, MA, Geller, B, Ryan, ND. The safety of desipramine (letter). *J Amer Acad Child Adolesc Psychiatry,* 1994;33:589-590.

Riddle, MA, Hardin, MT, Cho, SC, Woolston, JL, Leckman, JF. Desipramine treatment of boys with attention-deficit hyperactivity disorder and tics: Preliminary clinical experience. *J Amer Acad Child Adolesc Psychiatry,* 1988;27:811-814.

Riddle, MA, Nelson, JC, Kleinman, CS, Rasmusson, A, Leckman, JF, King, RA, Cohen, DJ. Sudden death in children receiving Norpramin: A review of three reported cases and commentary. *J Amer Acad Child Adolesc Psychiatry,* 1991; 30:104-108.

Ryan, ND. The pharmacologic treatment of child and adolescent depression. *Psych Clinic North Amer,* 1992;15:29-40.

Ryan, ND, Puig-Antich, J, Cooper, T, Rabinovich, H, Ambrosini, P, Davies, M, King, J, Torres, D, Fried, J. Imipramine in adolescent major depression: plasma level and clinical response. *Acta Psychiatr Scand,* 1986;73:275-288.

Ryan, ND, Puig-Antich, J, Cooper, TB, Rabinovich, H, Ambrosini, P, Fried, J, Davies, M, Torres, D, Suckow, RF. Relative safety of single versus divided dose imipramine in adolescent major depression. *J. Amer. Acad. Child Adolesc. Psychiatry* 1987; 26:400-406.

Saul, RC. Nortriptyline in attention deficit disorder. *Clin Neuropharmacol,* 1985; 8:382-384.

Schroeder, JS, Mullin, AV, Elliott, GR, Steiner, H, Nichols, M, Gordon, A, Paulos, M. Cardiovascular effects of desipramine in children. *J Amer Acad Child Adolesc Psychiatry,* 1989;28:376-379.

Shaefer, MS, Edmunds, AL, Markin, RS, Wood, P, Pillen J, Shaw, BW. Hepatic failure associated with imipramine therapy. *Pharmacotherapy,* 1990;10:66-69.

Spencer, T, Biederman, J, Wright, V, Danon, M. Growth deficits in children treated with desipramine: A controlled study. *J Amer Acad Child Adolesc Psychiatry,* 1992;31:235-243.

Spencer, T, Biederman, J, Kerman, K, Steingard, R, Wilens, T. Desipramine treatment of children with attention-deficit hyperactivity disorder and tic disorder or Tourette's syndrome. *J Amer Acad Child Adolesc Psychiatry,* 1993a;32: 354-360.

Spencer, T, Biederman, J, Wilens, T, Steingard, R, Geist, D. Nortriptyline treatment of children with attention-deficit hyperactivity disorder and tic disorder or Tourette's syndrome. *J Amer Acad Child Adolesc Psychiatry,* 1993b; 32:205-210.

Squires, LA, Neumeyer, AM, Bloomberg, J, Krishnamovsthy, KS. Hyperpyrexia in an adolescent on desipramine treatment. *Clin Pediatr,* 1992;31:635-636.

Stept, ME, Subramony, SH. Peripheral neuropathy associated with protriptyline. *J Amer Acad Child Adolesc Psychiatry,* 1988;27:377-380.

Strober, M. The pharmacotherapy of depressive illness in adolescence: III. Diagnostic and conceptual issues in studies of tricyclic antidepressants. *J Child Adolesc Psychopharmacol,* 1992;2:23-29.

Tingelstad, JB. The cardiotoxicity of the tricyclics. *J Amer Acad Child Adolesc Psychiatry,* 1991;30:845-855.

United States Pharmacopeia, Drug Information, 1994, Volumes I and II. Sections on tricyclic antidepressants.

Wagner, KD, Fershtman, M. Potential mechanism of desipramine-related sudden death in children. *Psychosomatics,* 1993;34:8083.

Werry, JS. The safety of desipramine (letter). *J Amer Acad Child Adolesc Psychiatry,* 1994;33:588-589.

Wilens, TE, Beiderman, J, Spencer, T, Geist, DE. A retrospective study of serum levels and electrocardiographic effects of nortriptyline in children and adolescents. *J Amer Acad Child Adolesc Psychiatry,* 1993c;32:270-277.

Wilens, TE, Biederman, J, Geist, DE, Steingard, R, Spencer, T. Nortriptyline in the treatment of ADHD: A chart review of 58 cases. *J Amer Acad Child Adolesc Psychiatry,* 1993a;32:343-349.

Wilens, TE, Biederman, J, Baldessarini, RJ, Puopolo, PR, Flood, JG. Electrocardiographic effects of desipramine and 2-hydroxydesipramine in children, adolescents and adults treated with desipramine. *J Amer Acad Child Adolesc Psychiatry,* 1993b;32:798-804.

Winsberg, BG, Goldstein, S, Yepes, LE, Perel, JM. Imipramine and electrocardiographic abnormalities in hyperactive children. *Amer J Psych* 1975;132: 542-545.

Bupropion

Bloomingdale, LM. Change from Mg Pemoline to Bupropion in a 12-year-old boy, with attention-deficit hyperactivity disorder (letter). *J Clin Psychopharmacol,* 1990;10:382-383.

Burroughs Wellcome. Wellbutrin® product information, drug information division, personal communication.

Cardinale, VA (ed). *1994 Drug Topics Redbook,* Medical Economics Company, Inc, 1994;413.

Casat, CD, Pleasants, DZ, Van Wyck Fleet, J. A double-blind trial of bupropion in children with attention deficit disorder. *Psychopharmacol Bull,* 1987;23: 120-122.

Clay, TH, Gualtieri, CT, Evans, RW, Gullion, CM. Clinical and neuropsychological effects of the novel antidepressant bupropion. *Psychopharmacol Bull,* 1988;24:143-148.

Davidson, J. Seizures and bupropion: A review. *J Clin Psychiatry,* 1989;50: 256-261.

Horne, RL, Ferguson, JM, Pope, HG, Hudon, JI, Lineberry, CG, Ascher, J, Cato, A. Treatment of bulimia with bupropion: A multicenter controlled trial. *J Clin Psychiatry,* 1988;49:262-266.

Johnston, JA, Lineberry, CG, Ascher, JA, Davidson, J, Khayrallah, MA, Feighner, JP, Stark, P. A 102 center prospective study of seizure in association with bupropion. *J Clin Psychiatry,* 1991;52:450-456.

Physician's Desk Reference. Oradell, NJ. Medical Economic Data, 1994.

Simeon, JG, Ferguson, HB, Van Wyck Fleet, J. Bupropion effects in attention deficit and conduct disorders. *Can J Psych,* 1986;31:581-585.

Spencer, T, Biederman, J, Steingard, R, Wilens, T. Bupropion exacerbates tics in children with attention-deficit hyperactivity disorder and Tourette's syndrome. *J Am Acad Child Adolesc Psychiatry,* 1993;32:211-214.

United States Pharmacopeia, Drug Information, 1994, Volumes I and II. Sections on bupropion.

Monoamine Oxidase Inhibitors

Cardinale, VA (ed). *1994 Drug Topics Redbook,* Medical Economics Company, Inc., 1994;289,310.

Ryan, ND, Puig-Antich, J, Rabinovich, H, Fried, J, Ambrosini, P, Meyer, V, Torres, D, Dachille, S, Mazzie, D. MAOIs in adolescent major depression unresponsive to tricyclic antidepressants. *J Am Acad Child Adolesc Psychiatry,* 1988;27:755-758.

United States Pharmacopeia, Drug Information, 1994, Volumes I and II. Sections on monoamine oxidase inhibitors.

Zametkin, A, Rapoport, JL, Murphy, DL, Linnoila, M, Ismond, D. Treatment of hyperactive children with monoamine oxidase inhibitors. I. Clinical efficacy. *Arch Gen Psych,* 1985;42:962-966.

Selective Serotonin Reuptake Blockers

Achamallah, N, Decker, DH. Mania induced by fluoxetine in an adolescent patient. *Am J Psych,* 1991;148:1404.

Barrickman, L, Noyes, R, Kuperman, S, Schumacher, E, Verda, M. Treatment of ADHD with fluoxetine: A preliminary report. *J Amer Acad Child Adolesc Psychiatry,* 1991; 30:762-767.

Boulos, C, Kutcher, S, Gardner, D, Young, E. An open naturalistic trial of fluoxetine in adolescents and young adults with treatment-resistant major depression. *J Child Adolesc Psychopharmacology,* 1992;2:103-111.

Cardinale, VA (ed). *1994 Drug Topics Redbook,* Medical Economics Company, Inc., 1994;348.

Como, PG, Kurlan, R. An open-label trial of fluoxetine for obsessive-compulsive disorder in Gilles de la Tourette's syndrome. *Neurology,* 1991;41:872-874.

Cook, EH, Rowlett, R, Jaselskis, C, Leventhal, BL. Fluoxetine treatment of children and adults with autistic disorder and mental retardation. *J Amer Acad Child Adolesc Psychiatry,* 1992;31:739-745.

DeMaso, DR, Hunter, TA. Combining fluoxetine with desipramine. *J Amer Acad Child Adolesc Psychiatry,* 1990;29:151.

Eisenhauer, G, Jermain, DM. Fluoxetine and tics in an adolescent. *Annal Pharmacotherapy,* 1993;27:725-726.

Ghaziuddin, M. Mania induced by sertraline in a prepubertal child. *Am J Psych,* 1994;151:944.

Hersh, CB, Sokol, MS, Pfeffer CR. Transient psychosis with fluoxetine. *J Amer Acad Child Adolesc Psychiatry,* 1991;30:851-852.

Iancu, J, Ratzoni, G, Weitzman, A, Apter, A. More fluoxetine experience. *J Amer Acad Child Adolesc Psychiatry,* 1992;31:755-756.

Jafri, AB. Fluoxetine side effects. *J Amer Acad Child Adolesc Psychiatry*, 1991;30:852.

Jain, U, Birmaher, B, Garcia, M, Al-Shabbout, M, Ryan, N. Fluoxetine in children and adolescents with mood disorders: A chart review of efficacy and adverse effects. *J Child Adolesc Psychopharmacology*, 1992;2:259-265.

Jerome, L. Hypomania with fluoxetine. *J Amer Acad Child Adolesc Psychiatry*, 1991;30:850-851.

King, RA, Riddle, MA, Chappell, PB, Hardin, MT, Anderson, GM, Lombroso, P, Scahill, L. Emergence of self-destructive phenomena in children and adolescents during fluoxetine treatment. *J Amer Acad Child Adolesc Psychiatry*, 1991;30:179-186.

Kurlan, R, Como, PG, McDermott, M, McDermott, MP. A pilot controlled study of fluoxetine for obsessive-compulsive symptoms in children with Tourette's syndrome. *Clin Neuropharmacology*, 1993;16:167-172.

Liebowitz, MR, Hollander, E, Fairbanks, J, Campeas, R. Fluoxetine for adolescents with obsessive-compulsive disorder. *Am J Psych*, 1990;147:370-371.

Lyles, B, Sarkis, E, Kemph, JP. Fluoxetine and anorexia. *J Amer Acad Child Adolesc Psychiatry*, 1990;29:984-985.

March, JS, Moon, RL, Johnston, H. Fluoxetine-TCA interaction. *J Amer Acad Child Adolesc Psychiatry*, 1990;29:985-986.

Matthews, P, Quinn, D, Marcoux, GS, Falkenberg, K. Fluoxetine and neuroleptic synergistic effects. *J Amer Acad Child Adolesc Psychiatry*, 1991;30:154-155.

Physician's Desk Reference. Oradell, NJ: Medical Economic Data, 1994.

Riddle, MA, Hardin, MT, King, R, Scahill, L, Woolston, JL. Fluoxetine treatment of children and adolescents with Tourette's and obsessive compulsive disorders: Preliminary clinical experience. *J Amer Acad Child Adolesc Psychiatry*, 1990a,29:45-48.

Riddle, MA, Brown, N, Dzubinski, D, Jetmalani, AN, Law, Y, Woolston, JL. Fluoxetine overdose in an adolescent. *J Amer Acad Child Adolesc Psychiatry*, 1989;28:587-588.

Riddle, MA, King, RA, Hardin, MT, Scahill, L, Ort, SI, Chappell, P, Rasmusson, A, Leckman, JF, Cohen, DJ. Behavioral side effects of fluoxetine in children and adolescents. *J Child Adolesc Psychopharmacol*, 1990/1991; 1:193-198.

Riddle, MA, Scahill, L, King, RA, Hardin, MT, Anderson, GM, Ort, SI, Smith, JC, Leckman, JF, Cohen, DJ. Double-blind crossover trial of fluoxetine and placebo in children and adolescents with obsessive-compulsive disorder. *J Amer Acad Child Adolesc Psychiatry*, 1992;31:1062-1069.

Rosenberg, DR, Johnson, K, Sahl, R. Evolving mania in an adolescent treated with low-dose fluoxetine. *J Child Adolesc Psychopharmacology*, 1992;2:299-306.

Simeon, JG, Dinicola, VF, Ferguson, B, Copping, W. Adolescent depression: A placebo-controlled fluoxetine treatment study and follow-up. *Prog Neuro Psychopharmacol and Biol Psychiat*, 1990;14:791-795.

Venkataraman, S, Naylor, MW, King, CA. Mania associated with fluoxetine treatment in adolescents. *J Amer Acad Child Adolesc Psychiatry*, 1992;31:276-281.

United States Pharmacopeia, Drug Information, 1994, Volumes I and II. Sections on fluoxetine.

Walter, AM. Sympathomimetic-fluoxetine interaction. *J Amer Acad Child Adolesc Psychiatry,* 1992;31:565-566.

Trazodone

Cardinale, VA (ed). *1994 Drug Topics Redbook,* Medical Economics Company, Inc., 1994;161,391.

Fras, I. Trazodone and violence. *J Am Acad Child Adolesc Psychiatry,* 1987; 26:453.

Ghaziuddin, N, Alessi, NE. An open trial of trazodone in aggressive children. *J Child Adolesc Psychopharmacology,* 1992;2:291-297.

Physician's Desk Reference. Oradell, NJ: Medical Economic Data, 1994.

Thompson, JW, Ware, MR, Blashfield, RK. Psychotropic medication and priapism: A comprehensive review. *J Clin Psychiatry,* 1990;51:430-433.

United States Pharmacopeia, Drug Information, 1994, Volumes I and II. Sections on trazodone.

Zubieta, JK, Alessi, NE. Acute and chronic administration of trazodone in the treatment of disruptive behavior disorder in children. *J Clin Psychopharmacology,* 1992;12:346-351.

Chapter 3

Antipsychotics

Chlorpromazine hydrochloride
> Thorazine® is marketed by SmithKline French.
> Chlorpromazine is also available as a generic product.

Clozapine
> Clozaril® is marketed by Sandoz Pharmaceuticals.

Fluphenazine hydrochloride
> Prolixin® is marketed by Bristol-Myers Squibb.
> Permitil® is marketed by Schering.
> Fluphenazine is also available in generic form.

Haloperidol
> Haldol® is marketed by McNeil Pharmaceuticals.
> Haloperidol is also available in generic form.

Loxapine
> Loxitane® is marketed by Lederle Laboratories.

Mesoridazine
> Serentil® is marketed by Boehringer Ingleheim.

Molindone
> Moban® is marketed by DuPont Pharmaceuticals.

Pimozide

   Orap® is marketed by Lemmon Pharmaceuticals.

Thioridazine

   Mellaril® is marketed by Sandoz Pharmaceuticals.

   Thioridazine is available in generic form.

Thiothixene

   Navane® is marketed by Roerig Pharmaceuticals.

   Thiothixene is also available in generic form.

DSM-IV INDICATIONS

Autism (?)

Tourette's syndrome (?)

Schizophrenia (??)

Conduct disorder, aggression (???)

   FDA: Most of the antipsychotics are not indicated for children less than 12 years of age. Exceptions include: clozapine and loxapine are not indicated in adolescents less than 16 years of age; haloperidol is not indicated for children less than three years of age; thioridazine is not indicated for children less than two years of age; chlorpromazine is not indicated for children less than six months, and fluphenazine is unspecified (*PDR,* 1994).

   USP: Children appear to be prone to develop neuromuscular or extrapyramidal reactions, especially dystonias, and should be closely monitored while receiving these agents (*USPDI,* 1994).

CONTRAINDICATIONS: Hypersensitivity to an agent or class of agents (e.g., phenothiazines); tardive dyskinesia; neuroleptic malignant syndrome; hepatic or renal impairment; acute physical illnesses, dehydration, hyperpyrexia; for clozapine, concurrent use with agents that suppress bone marrow function; for the Prolixin® products, tartrazine sensitivity.

PHARMACOLOGY: The standard antipsychotics (excluding clozapine) are dopamine antagonists and are also referred to as neuroleptics. The antipsychotics are used for a variety of psychotic disorders in adults. Antipsychotics will decrease the positive symptoms of schizophrenia (hallucinations, delusion, and formal thought disorders), but do not change or may worsen negative symptoms of schizophrenia (apathy and anergia). Blockade of dopamine in the nigrostriatal pathway leads to extrapyramidal symptoms of pseudoparkinsonism, dystonias, and akathisia. Long-term blockade may produce tardive dyskinesia. The potency of the antipsychotics is based on the affinity and binding of the drug to the dopamine-2 receptor and indicates the dose of a drug required to produce a particular effect. High doses of a low potency drug are required to produce the same effect as low doses of a high potency drug (Whitaker and Rao, 1992). For the standard antipsychotics, the low potency agents include chlorpromazine, thioridazine, and mesoridazine. Moderate potency antipsychotics include loxapine and molindone, and the high potency antipsychotics include fluphenazine, haloperidol, pimozide, and thiothixene. The efficacy of an agent may or may not be related to the potency and may be different for various disorders. Agents that have a phenothiazine chemical structure include chlorpromazine, thioridazine, mesoridazine, and fluphenazine.

The standard antipsychotics have numerous other pharmacological effects including anticholinergic, antihistaminergic and alphablocking effects. The anticholinergic effects of an antipsychotic are inversely related to the likelihood of extrapyramidal effects. Agents with high anticholinergic activity are less likely (but not absolutely) to cause extrapyramidal effects. The opposite is true for agents with low anticholinergic effects; these agents are more likely to cause extrapyramidal effects. The anticholinergic effects of the antipsychotics result in numerous adverse effects including blurred vision, dry mouth, urinary retention, constipation, sinus tachycardia, and memory dysfunction (Whitaker and Rao, 1992). Antipsychotic blockade of the histamine-1 receptor may result in sedation, weight gain, and hypotension. Antipsychotic blockade of the alpha-1 adrenergic receptor may result in postural hypotension, dizziness, and reflex tachycardia. Low potency agents (chlorpromazine, mesoridazine and thioridazine) have more anticholinergic, antihistaminergic, and alpha-blocking effects than high potency agents (fluphenazine, haloperidol, pimozide, and thiothixene). The efficacy of the standard antipsychotics is equivalent for groups of patients, so selection of an antipsychotic is based on indications, previous response, and the possibility of side effects.

Antagonism of dopamine activity in the tuburoinfundibular pathway produces elevated prolactin and may result in galactorrhea, gynecomastia, menstrual disturbances and a decrease in basal testosterone secretion (Apter et al., 1983). The long-term effects of hyperprolactinemia on psychosocial or physical development, or the effects of anticholinergic and antihistaminergic activity on cognitive development have not been investigated.

The atypical antipsychotic clozapine is a low potency, dibenzodiazepine that is used to treat patients with schizophrenia that have not responded to standard antipsychotic therapy. Clozapine produces a blockade of serotonin receptors and a selective dopamine blockade in the mesocortical and mesolimbic areas of the brain. Potentially clozapine has less dopamine blockade in the nigrostriatal tract, suggesting that clozapine may not cause tardive dyskinesia, but this is not definitive. Clozapine is associated with numerous adverse effects including agranulocytosis, seizures, and orthostatic hypotension.

STUDIES OF ANTIPSYCHOTIC EFFICACY

Autism

Campbell et al. (1978) reported a double-blind, placebo-controlled study of 40 children (aged 2.6 to 7.2 years) with autism. The results of this study indicate that haloperidol is more effective than placebo in treating hospitalized, preschool aged children. Improvement consisted of decreased levels of social withdrawal and stereotypes. Optimal doses of haloperidol were 0.5 to 4.0 mg/day. Side effects reported were excessive sedation, excitement, agitation, and acute dystonias. A follow-up study (Anderson et al., 1984) suggests that antipsychotics appear to be most effective in hyperactive children with autism, while behavioral problems in hypoactive autistic children seem to be exacerbated. An open pilot study assessed the efficacy of pimozide in hypoactive children with autism. This report suggests that pimozide (0.12 to 0.32 mg/kg/day) may decrease the hypoactivity of these children, however, one child became worse on pimozide (Ernst et al., 1992). In another open study of 12 children with pervasive developmental disorder, Joshi, Cappozzoli, and Coyle (1988) report that hyperactivity, aggression, and peer relationships improved on haloperidol or fluphenazine 0.04 mg/kg/day (less than 2 mg per day). Anderson et al. (1984) initially reported that haloperidol produces greater facilitation and retention of discriminate learning in the laboratory. These findings were not supported by a follow-up investigation; children with autism failed to learn on placebo or haloperidol (Anderson et al., 1989). However, there were no cognitive deficits observed with therapeutic doses of 0.5 to 4.0 mg per day.

In a double-blind study designed to determine the long-term efficacy of haloperidol in the treatment of autism, Perry et al. (1989) reported on 60 children treated with haloperidol for six months followed by an abrupt switch to a four-week placebo period. Patients (ages 2.3 to 7.9 years, mean 5.1 years) were included in the study if they responded to haloperidol and required further treatment. Patients were randomly assigned to continuous or discontinuous treatment with flexible doses of haloperidol. Discontinuous therapy consisted of five days of haloperidol followed by two days of placebo per week. Both regimens were equally effective in reducing the target symptoms of autism. As in the above studies, doses of haloperidol ranged from 0.5 to 4.0 mg/day (mean of 1.23 mg/day). During the four week placebo substitution, patients became worse during the first week. At the end of four weeks, 59 percent of the patients were rated as having mild to more severe deterioration in comparison to the treatment period. Forty-one percent of the patients were not rated as more severe during the four weeks of placebo (Perry et al., 1989). Children with prominent symptoms of irritability, angry, and labile affect and uncooperativeness were the best responders to haloperidol.

Patients in the above study were videotaped, prior to and after the six months of haloperidol, and each week during the four-week placebo trial (Campbell et al., 1988). Ratings for abnormal involuntary movements were done using the Abnormal Involuntary Movement Scale (AIMS) from the National Institutes of Mental Health. Dyskinesias were observed in 29.2 percent of patients. Of these patients, 20.8 percent had tardive dyskinesia and 79.2 percent had withdrawal dyskinesia. Withdrawal dyskinesia occurred between four and 34 days after drug withdrawal. The duration of dyskinetic movements varied from seven to 225 days. Dyskinetic movements were observed in the facial and oral area, the extremities, trunk, and one patient had laryngo-diaphragmatic movements. Campbell et al. (1988) reported that they found no irreversible tardive dyskinesia and suggest that the risk of sustained tardive dyskinesia in the child appears to be less than in adults. Campbell et al. (1983) report that normal children as well as children with infantile autism may exhibit abnormal, stereotypic behaviors. Bucco-lingual facial movements (lip puckering and tongue movements) were most frequently observed. In consideration of the high rate of withdrawal dyskinesias and the possibility of tardive dyskinesia, predrug and ongoing evaluations of movement disorders are essential for adequate monitoring of antipsychotic effects.

Tourette's Syndrome

The majority of patients with Tourette's syndrome do not require drug therapy. For those patients who are impaired by the intensity or frequency of the motor and vocal tics, haloperidol is the drug of choice. Pimozide is also effective, but is reserved for patients who do not tolerate haloperidol. Tourette's syndrome spontaneously goes through periods of exacerbation and improvement, and the symptoms may be voluntarily controlled for periods of time. Tourette's syndrome has a relatively high rate of placebo response, especially in long-term studies. The nature of this disorder makes it particularly difficult to assess the effects of drug therapy. In addition, the antipsychotics are associated with numerous acute and chronic extrapyramidal effects that may be indistinguishable from the symptoms of Tourette's syndrome (Bruun, 1984).

Controlled and open studies have reported the efficacy of the antipsychotics in the treatment of Tourette's (Shapiro and Shapiro, 1982; Shapiro and Shapiro, 1983; Shapiro and Shapiro, 1984; Singer, Gammon, and Quaskey, 1985-86). One controlled study has compared the efficacy of haloperidol and pimozide in a group of 57 patients aged eight to 46 years (Shapiro et al., 1989). Patients were randomly assigned to haloperidol, pimozide, or placebo. The mean daily dose of haloperidol was 4.5 mg/day (mean of 0.08 mg/kg/day) and 10.6 mg/day (mean of 0.18 mg/kg/day) for pimozide. Haloperidol was slightly more effective than pimozide but both drugs were more effective than placebo in reducing the frequency of tics. Adverse effects were not separated for children versus adults but included akinesia, akathisia, tremor, mask-like facies, depression, cognitive dulling, increased appetite, weight gain, difficulty urinating, and gynecomastia. The incidence of adverse effects were comparable between the two drugs.

Antipsychotics may induce a variety of behavioral and affective disturbances in children and adolescents with Tourette's syndrome. Bruun (1988) reported a retrospective chart review of 208 cases of Tourette's syndrome that were treated with low doses of haloperidol, pimozide, or fluphenazine. Thirty-four children developed dose-related symptoms of dysphoria or depression. Bruun (1988) described a "threshold dose" above which the patient would complain of dysphoria and below which the dysphoric symptoms were absent. The "threshold dose" varied by patient. The symptoms of dysphoria are crying spells, irritability, social withdrawal, anxiety, fearfulness, and a preoccupation with morbid subject matter. School phobias appeared in eight children. Bruun (1988) suggests that school phobia is related to antipsychotic-induced dysphoria.

Nine children developed akathisia with an apparent worsening in symptoms of Tourette's syndrome. These children typically improved on initial doses, but with further dose increases appeared to lose the positive effects of the medication. Four adolescents and one child developed hostility, irritability, and aggression. The patients became explosive and developed regressive behavior. Bruun (1988) suggests that these effects are manifestations of akathisia. In each of the above cases, a reduction in dose resolved the symptoms of dysphoria or akathisia. Three patients developed "fog states" during which the patients felt out of touch with, but not unaware of, their surroundings for minutes to hours at a time. One of these patients also developed psychomotor seizures. Two patients responded to primidone therapy, and one patient responded to discontinuation of the antipsychotic. Three patients developed abnormal involuntary movements that were distinguishable from the symptoms of Tourette's syndrome. In all three cases, haloperidol was discontinued and the dyskinesia resolved within weeks to months. Bruun (1988) suggests that the above side effects of the antipsychotics may be more apparent in patients with Tourette's syndrome, however the frequency of these effects in other patients has not been reported. Practitioners are encouraged to monitor for the above adverse effects and reduce the dose or discontinue the antipsychotic if necessary. Patients with Tourette's syndrome who do not experience intolerable side effects from the antipsychotics are able to perform on educational, intellectual, and neuropsychological tests at a level comparable to unmedicated patients with Tourette's syndrome (Bornstein and Yang, 1991).

Schizophrenia

Spencer et al. (1992) reported the preliminary results of the first double-blind, placebo-controlled trial investigating the efficacy of haloperidol in the treatment of children with schizophrenia. The presenting signs and symptoms of schizophrenia were auditory and visual hallucinations, delusions, thought disorders, and inappropriate affect. Patients, aged 5.5 to 11.75 years, were randomly assigned to receive four weeks of placebo followed by four weeks of haloperidol, or, alternatively, four weeks of haloperidol followed by four weeks of placebo. Haloperidol was superior to placebo for reducing the target symptoms of ideas of reference, hallucinations, persecutory, and other thinking disorders. The effects of haloperidol did not reach statistical significance for the targeted symptoms of suspicious or blunted affect, delusions, and peculiar fantasies. The optimal doses of haloperidol were 0.5 to 3.5 mg per day (0.02 to 0.12 mg/kg/day). For eight of the 12 patients, optimal doses of haloperidol were 0.04 to 0.06 mg/kg/day. The adverse effects of haloperidol were drowsiness, drooling, dizziness, mask-like facies, cogwheel rigidity, decreased arm-swing, mild tic-like lip movements, minimal vermicular tongue movements, tongue discomfort, and acute dystonic reactions. These side effects resolved with a reduction in the dose or with continued treatment. Acute dystonic reactions were treated with oral administration of 25 mg of diphenhydramine elixir.

Pool et al. (1976) reported the only randomized, double-blind, placebo-controlled, four-week study comparing the effectiveness of haloperidol and loxapine in 75 adolescents with schizophrenia. Haloperidol and loxapine were superior to placebo in controlling delusions, hallucinations, thought disorders, and social withdrawal. The average daily doses of haloperidol were 9.8 mg/day and loxapine 87.5 mg/day. Extrapyramidal effects, particularly muscle rigidity, and sedation were frequently reported in the patients on loxapine or haloperidol. Realmuto et al. (1984) reported a single-blind study of 21 adolescents with schizophrenia that were randomly assigned to four to six weeks of thioridazine or thiothixene. The symptoms of hallucinations, anxiety, tension, and excitement improved in 50 percent of the patients. Cognitive disorganization was minimally improved. The authors reported that despite improvements in symptoms, patients continued to be quite impaired. Extrapyramidal effects were more frequent with thiothixene therapy while dizziness and orthostatic hypotension were more frequent with thioridazine. Drowsiness accounted for 40 percent of all side effects and was more common with thioridazine therapy. The optimal therapeutic dose of thiothixene was 0.30 mg/kg/day (range of 4.8 to 42.6 mg/day), and 3.3 mg/kg/day for thioridazine (range of 91 to 228 mg/day). The authors suggest that the two antipsychotics were equally efficacious, but the high potency agents were associated with less sedation and may be preferred over the low potency agents for the treatment of adolescents with schizophrenia. Additional placebo-controlled trials conducted over a longer duration of time are needed in adolescents and children with schizophrenia.

There are numerous case studies using clozapine in the treatment of adolescents with schizophrenia (Birmaher et al., 1992; Blanz and Schmidt, 1993; Boxer and Davidson, 1992; Freedman et al., 1994; Frazier et al., 1994; Jacobsen et al., 1994; Levkovitch et al., 1994; Remschmidt et al., 1994; Towbin, Dykens, and Pugliese, 1994). In addition, there are four case reports of children aged ten to 12 years that successfully responded to clozapine (Mozes et al., 1994). There is no age limit for the Clozaril® Patient Management System. All reported patients were treatment resistant to standard antipsychotic therapies. The usual age range for adolescents in pharmacological studies is 13 to 17 years. The reports from Germany (Blanz and Schmidt, 1993) included patients as young as ten years old. The average daily dose of clozapine ranged from 240 to 370 mg per day with a range of 125 to 825 mg/day. Adverse effects that resulted in discontinuation of therapy were orthostatic hypotension, seizures, and leukopenia. Clozapine therapy was associated with hypersalivation, drowsiness, transient fever, weight gain, tachycardia, sedation, constipation, seizures, nausea, dizziness, leukopenia, elevation of liver enzymes, and extrapyramidal effects. Dose-related adverse effects were enuresis, sedation, and seizures. In the separate report by Mozes et al. (1994) four children were treated with 175 to 300 mg of clozapine and had side effects of hypersalivation, drowsiness, transient fever, enuresis, and excitatory changes on the electroencephalogram (EEG). The authors avoided further increases in dose if EEG changes were observed.

These initial reports suggest that clozapine may be effective in the treatment of child and adolescent schizophrenia. Slow and progressive improvements with clozapine therapy may occur over weeks to months, however, auditory hallucinations may be resistant to clozapine therapy. The positive symptoms of schizophrenia, delusions, hallucinations, thought disorders, and excitement are more responsive to clozapine therapy than are negative symptoms. The negative symptoms of schizophrenia include anhedonia, flattened affect and autistic behavior. Clozapine offers an alternative therapy to the standard antipsychotics. In addition, clozapine may not cause tardive dyskinesia, but this is not definitive. Further investigations and reports will indicate the relative risks and benefits of clozapine in the treatment of children and adolescents with schizophrenia.

Conduct Disorder

A pilot double-blind study by Campbell, Cohen, and Small (1982) included 15 children (ages six to 12 years, mean of 8.68 years) with aggressiveness, hyperactivity, and explosive behavior. The diagnoses of the patients included hyperkinetic reaction of childhood, unsocialized aggressive reaction of childhood, and schizophrenia childhood type (Campbell, Cohen, and Small, 1982). After a two-week placebo washout, patients were randomly assigned to haloperidol, chlorpromazine, or lithium. Haloperidol doses of 4 to 16 mg/day (mean of 9.2 mg/day), chlorpromazine doses of 100 to 200 mg/day (mean of 150 mg/day), and lithium doses of 1,250 to 2,000 mg/day were administered during the three week trial. Blood levels of lithium were maintained between 0.76 to 1.24 mEq/L. Side effects associated with lithium were insomnia, drowsiness, and one case of a toxic confusional state. Side effects associated with haloperidol were drowsiness, drooling, slurred speech, and dystonic reactions, and chlorpromazine was associated with drowsiness. All three drugs were effective in reducing aggressive behavior. The authors note that chlorpromazine therapy led to excessive drowsiness at relatively low doses (Campbell, Cohen, and Small, 1982).

A follow-up, double-blind, placebo-controlled study, of 61 children, aged 5.2 to 12.9 years (mean of 8.97 years) assessed the efficacy of haloperidol and lithium carbonate (Campbell et al., 1984; Platt et al., 1984). Lithium and haloperidol were used for their anti-aggressive, but non-sedative properties. Patients were diagnosed with undersocialized, aggressive conduct disorder, and were unresponsive to various outpatient treatments. The patients did not take any concurrent medications, were in good physical health, and were not mentally retarded. The optimal dose of haloperidol was 1 to 6 mg/day (mean of 2.95 mg/day) or 0.04 to 0.21 mg/kg/day (mean of 0.096 mg/kg/day). The optimal dose of lithium was 500 to 2,000 mg/day (mean of 1,166 mg/day) that resulted in lithium blood levels of 0.32 to 1.51 mEq/L (mean of 0.993 mEq/L). The side effects of haloperidol were excessive sedation, acute dystonic reaction, and drooling. The side effects of lithium were stomachache, headache, and tremor of the hands. Electroencephalograms (EEG) were obtained in 48 of the patients at baseline, and 58 percent of these patients had an abnormal EEG. Haloperidol or lithium therapy was associated with a worsening of the EEG parameters with paroxysmal or focal abnormalities at optimal treatment doses (Bennett et al., 1983). Haloperidol and lithium were superior to the effects of placebo in reducing aggression, hostility, and hyperactivity. The staff treating these patients indicated that patients taking lithium showed the greatest improvement; lithium was also associated with less sedation. Haloperidol was associated with mild negative effects on cognition. The authors indicated that although the effects of haloperidol on cognition were mild, any negative effect is undesirable, particularly for children with academic difficulties (Platt et al., 1984).

DEVELOPMENTAL PHARMACOKINETICS

(The pharmacokinetics of these agents have not been fully investigated in children and adolescents.)

Absorption: In adults, peak plasma levels occur within two to four hours. Oral liquid forms are absorbed faster than tablets or capsules.

Metabolism: Children appear to metabolize haloperidol faster than adults, but children appear to more sensitive to the therapeutic and adverse effects. This suggests that lower doses are indicated. In general, the antipsychotics are extensively metabolized to numerous active and inactive metabolites.

Half-life: The half-lives for most agents have not been investigated in children or adolescents. Sallee et al. (1987) reported the average half-life of pimozide in five children with Tourette's as 66 hours with a wide range of 24 to 142 hours.

Plasma levels: Administering a fixed dose per day of haloperidol results in a wide variance in steady-state plasma concentrations. At a given mg/kg daily dose of haloperidol, the plasma concentrations may vary up to 15 fold (Morselli et al., 1979). Within each patient, the haloperidol dose to plasma level ratio is more consistent. Morselli, Bianchetti, and Dugas (1983) suggest that in the treatment of psychosis, children are more likely to show a positive response to haloperidol levels of 6 to 10 ng/ml. Patients with Tourette's syndrome require much lower haloperidol plasma levels of 0.5 to 4 ng/ml. Different disorders may require different plasma concentrations, and dosage should be titrated on the basis of response and adverse effects. Adverse effects are more frequent at higher haloperidol plasma levels. Other antipsychotic plasma levels have not been studied in children and adolescents (or adults).

DOSAGE RANGES

It is recommended that doses of antipsychotics be started low and increased slowly to avoid side effects. Children appear to be very sensitive to the effects of the antipsychotics and do not require higher doses on a weight basis. There is a large variability in plasma levels to a fixed dose and practitioners are encouraged to titrate the dose to the individual patient response. For patients that have an initial response and then become worse, dose reduction is indicated. Some patients will respond to very low doses and steady-state plasma levels may not occur for several days. The suggested dosage ranges below are based on a very limited number of patients reported.

Autism: Initial doses of haloperidol are 0.25 mg once or twice daily increasing by 0.25 mg per week. Maximal doses are 0.5 to 4 mg per day in divided doses. Slow dosage increases appear to decrease the likelihood of extrapyramidal symptoms (Campbell et al., 1978). Pimozide doses of 0.12 to 0.32 mg/kg/day (Ernst et al., 1992) and fluphenazine doses of 0.04 mg/kg/day (Joshi, Capozzoli, and Coyle, 1988) have been utilized.

Tourette's Syndrome: Optimal doses of haloperidol 0.08 mg/kg/day or pimozide 0.18 mg/kg/day have been reported (Shapiro et al., 1989).

Schizophrenia:

Children: Haloperidol doses of 0.02 to 0.12 mg/kg/day have been reported (Spencer et al., 1992).

Adolescents: Average daily doses of haloperidol 9.8 mg, loxitane doses of 87.5 mg (Poole et al., 1976), thiothixene doses of 0.30 mg/kg/day, and thioridazine doses of 3.3 mg/kg/day (Realmuto et al., 1984) have been reported. Clozapine doses vary from 125 to 825 mg per day with an average of 300 mg per day.

ADVERSE EFFECTS REPORTED IN CHILDREN AND ADOLESCENTS

COMMON

Early onset of extrapyramidal effects (akathisia, dystonia, and pseudoparkinsons) are more likely with high potency than low potency antipsychotics. Sedation, anticholinergic effects, and cardiovascular effects are more likely with low potency than high potency antipsychotics.

Dry mouth: Sucking on bits of ice or drinking water may help this anticholinergic side effect. If the patient chooses to suck on hard candy or chew gum frequently the sugarless variety is indicated. A dry mouth and sugar may result in a candida infection or damage to the teeth.

Drooling or hypersalivation: This adverse effect is reported with the standard antipsychotics, but is frequently reported with clozapine. Benztropine therapy may be indicated for adolescents (Boxer and Davidson, 1992).

Constipation: This anticholinergic side effect may be reduced by encouraging the patient to drink plenty of water, and eat more vegetables, fruits, and bran. If indicated, a mild stool softener should be routinely administered.

Sedation: Low potency antipsychotics (chlorpromazine, clozapine, mesoridazine, molindone) frequently cause this side effect, but even high potency antipsychotics may cause this reaction in children or adolescents (Whitaker and Rao, 1992). Sedation is an unacceptable side effect that inhibits learning and social functioning. Sedation may be alleviated by reducing the dose or changing to a low dose of a high potency antipsychotic.

Fatigue: Decreased energy or easy fatiguability may occur in the absence of sedation. Fatigue may also be associated with decreased hepatic function and leukopenia. Appropriate laboratory tests may be necessary if this side effect does not respond to dose reduction.

Cognitive functioning: The specific effects of the antipsychotics on learning have not been adequately assessed. The anticholinergic and sedative effects of the antipsychotics may have a negative effect on cognitive function. Platt et al. (1984) found that haloperidol had a mild negative effect on cognitive functioning in children with aggressive behavior. The effects of the antipsychotics on cognitive functioning may be dose related, and dose reduction may be indicated.

Akathisia: The symptoms of akathisia are not well formulated in children. This reaction may consist of restlessness and agitation and can be easily misidentified as a worsening of symptoms or hyperactivity (Bruun, 1988; Weiden and Bruun, 1987). When a child initially responds but with continued therapy worsens, the patient may have akathisia. Akathisia is associated with higher doses of antipsychotics, and dosage reduction is the indicated. There are preliminary reports of patients with akathisia that responded to propranolol (Chandler, 1990) or clonazepam (Kutcher et al., 1987; Kutcher et al., 1989) therapy.

Pseudoparkinsons: The manifestations of pseudoparkinsons include tremor, rigidity, bradykinesia, drooling, and mask-like face. Pseudoparkinsonism occurs more often in children five years of age and older and is rarely found in preschool children. Dosage reduction is indicated, and anticholinergic drugs (e.g., benztropine or diphenhydramine) are not recommended for children (Campbell, 1985). An anticholinergic medication may be indicated in adolescents with pseudoparkinsons (Keepers, Clappison, and Casey, 1983).

Photosensitivity: Antipsychotics are secreted into the skin and increase the chance of severe sunburn. All patients must wear a sunscreen lotion and protective clothing when outside to avoid the dangers of this side effect.

Hypotension: Postural hypotension may be relieved by administering the medication in divided doses. Patients may develop a tolerance to this effect. Patients should be warned not to get up too quickly from a lying or sitting position. Dosage reduction may be indicated. For severe cases of hypotension, the patient should be placed in a horizontal position with the feet raised, and intravenous, isotonic fluids may be indicated. The use of an alpha and beta stimulant (e.g., epinephrine) or a beta stimulant (e.g., isoproterenol) is contraindicated. An alpha stimulant (e.g., norepinephrine) may be indicated. Subsequent dose reduction or discontinuation of the antipsychotic is indicated.

LESS COMMON

Dystonia: A dystonic reaction is an acute, involuntary, striated muscle spasm. A dystonic reaction occurs within the first few days of therapy after initiating therapy, increasing the dose, or switching to a higher potency agent. Torticollis, opisthotonos, oculogyric crisis, and spasms of the tongue or jaw are the most common forms of dystonia. A dystonic reaction to one antipsychotic suggests a susceptibility to dystonias with other antipsychotics (Ernst, Gonzalez, and Campbell, 1993). All dystonic reactions require medical attention, but rarely are life threatening with the exception of a laryngeal dystonia. A laryngeal dystonia may result in compromised respiratory function and possibly death if not treated immediately. Dystonic reactions are more common with high potency than low potency antipsychotics. Researchers have used a single oral or injectable dose of diphenhydramine 25 mg to relieve a dystonic reaction (Campbell et al., 1984). Potentially, the prophylactic use of anticholinergic agents for adolescents reduces the risk of dystonia and other extrapyramidal effects (Keepers, Clappison, and Casey, 1983; Sramek et al., 1986). However, practitioners do not routinely prescribe anticholinergic agents unless extrapyramidal symptoms develop.

Antipsychotic-induced catatonia: Muscle rigidity, mutism, and staring may be an early stage in the progression of neuroleptic malignant syndrome. Immediate discontinuation of the antipsychotic agent and initiation of a benzodiazepine is recommended (Woodbury and Woodbury, 1992).

Neuroleptic Malignant Syndrome: The signs and symptoms of neuroleptic malignant syndrome (NMS) include hyperthermia, altered consciousness, autonomic instability (tachycardia, labile hypotension, diaphoresis, pallor), lead pipe muscular rigidity, tachycardia, hypertension, elevated levels of creatinine phosphate kinase (CPK), staring and mutism (Latz and McCracken, 1992; Steingard et al., 1992). If not treated, NMS can proceed to coma and death. Both high and low potency antipsychotics are associated with NMS. Conservative treatment includes discontinuation of the antipsychotic, hospitalization, and possible administration of bromocriptine (Diamond and Hayes, 1986; Joshi, Capozzoli, and Coyle, 1991; Merry et al., 1986; Tenenbein, 1985/86). Joshi, Capozzoli, and Coyle (1991) suggest affective disorders may be a risk factor for the development of this side effect. Rechallenge with an antipsychotic may result in a recurrence of NMS.

Tardive dyskinesia: This side effect has been reported in children within 3.5 months of antipsychotic initiation. The manifestations of tardive dyskinesia are abnormal involuntary movements of any striated muscle including muscles of the face, jaw, neck, upper and lower extremities, fingers, toes, and trunk. The movements are usually rhythmical, but may be athetotic or tic-like (Campbell et al., 1983). The movements may be difficult to distinguish from symptoms of Tourette's syndrome (Silva, Magee, and Friedhoff, 1993a). Tardive dyskinesia needs to be differentiated from withdrawal dyskinesia which occurs upon antipsychotic withdrawal or dose reduction. Withdrawal dyskinesia occurs within 14 days after neuroleptic discontinuation, and depending upon the neuroleptic exposure, the signs and symptoms are usually reversible. A baseline assessment of abnormal movements and stereotypies is necessary in monitoring for signs and symptoms of tardive dyskinesia (Campbell et al., 1983; Meiselas et al., 1989). Based on preliminary findings, withdrawal dyskinesia is more common in children than maintenance-onset tardive dyskinesia and most dyskinesias in this age group are reversible (Campbell et al., 1988). However, sustained dyskinetic movements have been reported (Gualtieri and Patterson, 1986; Karagianis and Nagpurkar, 1990; Riddle et al., 1987). There is no known treatment for tardive dyskinesia. Discontinuation of the neuroleptic is indicated. Anticholinergics drugs may worsen the symptoms.

Tics: Abnormal tic-like movements have been reported following short-term (ten days) of antipsychotic therapy that resolved with discontinuation of the antipsychotic

(Gualtieri and Patterson, 1986). Long-term (three years) administration of haloperidol 3 mg/day has also resulted in tic-like movements after withdrawal of the antipsychotic (Perry, Nobler, and Campbell, 1989).

Memory impairment: There are no studies of cognitive changes with antipsychotics, however there is a potential for this side effect due to sedation and anticholinergic effects. This effect needs further evaluation (McClellan and Werry, 1992).

Anxiety, depression, or dysphoria: School avoidance, social phobia, separation anxiety, and anxiety have been reported in patients with Tourette's syndrome who are taking antipsychotics. Symptoms remit after reducing the dose or discontinuing the antipsychotic (Bruun, 1988; Linet, 1985; Mikkelsen, Detlor, and Cohen, 1981).

Behavioral toxicity: Exacerbations in behavior may be attributed to akathisia. Irritability and temper tantrums may occur and respond to dosage reductions.

Delirium: Antipsychotics can induce central anticholinergic toxicity that is manifested by confusion, disorientation, irritability, aggressiveness, and visual hallucinations. Discontinuation of the antipsychotic is indicated. Reinitiation at a lower dose or switching to a higher potency, lower anticholinergic antipsychotic is suggested.

Weight gain: The antihistaminergic effects of the standard antipsychotics may increase the appetite and result in excessive weight gain. This side effect has not been fully evaluated in the pediatric population (Silva et al., 1993b). Appropriate diet and exercise regimens are indicated. Clozapine therapy may also be associated with weight gain.

Enuresis: Campbell (1985) indicates that enuresis may be avoided by administering the dose in the morning or late afternoon, avoiding a bedtime dose. For clozapine, a reduction in the dose may alleviate this side effect.

Urinary retention: Urinary retention is an anticholinergic effect that may require discontinuation of the drug. Bethanechol, a peripheral cholinesterase inhibitor, has been used in adults to treat this side effect.

Hepatic dysfunction: The incidence of cholestatic jaundice is unknown in children and adolescents. Liver function tests are indicated at baseline and repeated if symptoms of nausea, vomiting, fatigue, and yellow eyes or skin develop.

Hematological effects: Agranulocytosis has been reported in adults. For the standard antipsychotics a baseline complete blood count (CBC) with differential is indicated. A follow-up CBC with differential is indicated if the patient develops a fever, fatigue, sore throat, or other infection. Clozapine therapy requires a weekly white blood count with differential as part of the Clozaril® Patient Management System.

Seizures: Antipsychotics reduce the seizure threshold and may induce seizures. Patients who develop seizures or have a known seizure history require anticonvulsant therapy. Clozapine-induced seizures appear to be dose related and may respond to dose reduction (Freedman et al., 1994).

Cardiac arrthymias: Increased heart rate, prolongation of the QT and PR intervals and T wave, and depression of the ST segment are more commonly associated with the low potency antipsychotics (chlorpromazine, mesoridazine, and thioridazine), but occasionally are found in patients taking moderate or high potency antipsychotics (Whitaker and Rao, 1992). Pimozide produces ECG changes in up to 25 percent of patients treated for Tourette's syndrome and appears to be dose related. Pimozide should be discontinued if T-wave inversion or U waves occur. The dose of pimozide should not be increased if there is significant prolongation of the corrected Q-T interval. Unlike the other standard antipsychotics pimozide has calcium-channel-blocking properties and may produce bradycardia (*see* Monitoring Guidelines).

Pigmentary retinopathy: This adverse effect is associated with thioridazine therapy in excess of 800 mg per day in adults. The maximum adult total daily dose of thiorida-zine is 800 mg. For children, ages two to 12 years, the manufacturer suggests a maximum dose of thioridazine 3 mg/kg/day.

Hyperprolactinemia: An increase in prolactin levels may re-sult in gynecomastia, galactorrhea, irregular menstrua-tion, or amenorrhea. In adults, the administration of a dopamine agonist (bromocriptine) reduces these side ef-fects. Cautious administration of low dose bromocriptine is suggested (Teicher and Glod, 1990). Clozapine may not increase prolactin blood levels (Gonzalez and Micha-nie, 1992).

Sexual dysfunction: Impotence, delayed ejaculation, or retro-grade ejaculation may occur.

ALLERGIC REACTION: The most common allergic reac-tion consists of a maculopapular rash on the face, neck, or upper chest and extremities.

TOXICITY: The manifestations of overdose may include central nervous system depression, hypotension, extrapy-ramidal reactions, agitation, delirium, seizures, fever, hy-pothermia, and cardiac arrhythmias.

DRUG INTERACTIONS

DRUG	DRUGS	EFFECT
Antipsy-chotics	Anticholinergic agents	Combination therapy results in enhanced peripheral and central anticholinergic effects (*see* Ad-verse Effects, Delirium). Admin-istration of anticholinergic agents may decrease the absorption of the antipsychotics. Symptoms of tardive dyskinesia may worsen with anticholinergic therapy.
Antipsy-chotics	Tricyclic antidepressants	Tricyclic antidepressant and anti-psychotic serum concentrations

		may be increased. Anticholinergic, sedative, and cardiovascular adverse effects may be increased.
Antipsychotics	Fluoxetine	Extrapyramidal effects may be increased. Fluoxetine may inhibit the metabolism of the antipsychotics, resulting in higher antipsychotic blood levels.
Antipsychotics	Lithium	Concurrent use may mask the early signs of lithium toxicity (nausea, vomiting). Concurrent use may also result in neurotoxicity, seizures, or neuroleptic malignant syndrome, even in the presence of therapeutic lithium and antipsychotic doses and blood levels.
Antipsychotics	Aluminum salts, Antacids, Antidiarrheals	Administer antacids two hours apart from antipsychotics. Concurrent administration will result in decreased absorption of the antipsychotics.
Antipsychotics	Stimulants	Concurrent administration will decrease the effectiveness of both agents.
Antipsychotics	Valprioc acid, Phenytoin	Alterations in serum levels have occurred and monitoring of the serum levels is indicated.
Antipsychotics	Carbamazepine	Decreased haloperidol levels have occurred.
Antipsychotics	Barbiturates	Barbiturates may reduce antipsychotic plasma levels.
Antipsychotics	Propranolol	Increased plasma levels of both drugs may occur. Hypotension may be more pronounced.

Antipsychotics	Epinephrine	Concurrent administration is contraindicated.
Antipsychotics	Alcohol	Alcohol will add to the sedative effects of the antipsychotics.
Antipsychotics	Tobacco smoking	Concurrent use may increase metabolism resulting in decreased blood levels of antipsychotics.
Clozapine	Drugs that may cause agranulocytosis including antibiotics, anticonvulsants, antihistamines, psychotropics, etc.	There are numerous drugs that are associated with agranulocytosis and are contraindicated during clozapine therapy. The extensive list of drug interactions is available from the Clozaril® Patient Management System. If possible, avoid concurrent medications during clozapine therapy. If concurrent medications are necessary, more intensive monitoring for bone marrow suppression and signs of infection are indicated.

MONITORING GUIDELINES

Baseline Assessment:

- History and physical, including weight and height of the patient.
- Laboratory evaluations including liver function tests and a complete blood count with differential.
- Orthostatic blood pressures and pulse should be obtained.
- An electrocardiogram is indicated if the lower potency antipsychotics (thioridazine, chlorpromazine, and mesoridazine) or pimozide are used (Sylvester, 1993), or if there is history of cardiac problems.
- An electroencephalogram is indicated prior to clozapine therapy (Blanz and Schmidt, 1993; Freedman et al., 1994), and in patients with a possible history of seizures (all antipsychotics).

- A thorough explanation of the risks and benefits of antipsychotic drug therapy should be presented to the patient and family. Informed consent should be obtained from parents or guardians prior to initiation of drug therapy. If possible, assent should be obtained from those patients under legal age of consent. If the psychotic state prevents giving assent, then treatment may be initiated and assent obtained after the patient has improved sufficiently to do so (McClellan and Werry, 1992).
- Baseline assessment of targeted symptoms is needed to accurately monitor the effects of the antipsychotic.
- Baseline assessment of involuntary or abnormal movements is necessary to monitor for extrapyramidal adverse effects.

Time Pattern for Response:

- In the treatment of schizophrenia, a four to six week trial is necessary to determine if the drug is effective or not (Campbell et al., 1988; McClellan and Werry, 1992). If efficacy is not apparent after this time period, a different antipsychotic is indicated (McClellan and Werry, 1992).

Follow-Up Assessment:

- Blood pressure and pulse should routinely be obtained during dose titration and during follow-up.
- For pimozide, an electrocardiogram is indicated during dosage titration and as indicated by patient status (Shapiro and Shapiro, 1984). Any indication of prolongation of the QT-corrected interval beyond an absolute limit of 0.47 seconds for children, or more than a 25 percent increase above the patient's original baseline should be considered a basis for stopping further dosage increases and possible dose reduction.
- Liver function tests and complete blood counts with differentials are suggested according to patient status.
- Patients in the Clozaril® Patient Management System require weekly white blood cell counts with differential. The Clozaril® Patient Management System specifies

continued treatment or discontinuation according to the white blood cell count.
- Monitor for extrapyramidal effects. A formal assessment for tardive dyskinesia should occur every three months. There are several assessment scales including the Abnormal Involuntary Movement Scale (National Institutes of Mental Health, 1985) and the Dyskinesia Identification System: Condensed User Scale (Sprague and Kalachnik, 1991).
- For the treatment of schizophrenia, the drug is continued for four to six months followed by dose reduction and discontinuation to allow for reassessment of the need for continued drug therapy (Campbell et al., 1988). Prolonged use should be avoided due to the significant risk of tardive dyskinesia and neuroleptic malignant syndrome.

Drug Discontinuation:

- Taper the dose of the antipsychotic to minimize symptoms of withdrawal that include nightmares, insomnia, increased salivation, nausea, severe vomiting (Grob, 1986; Yepes and Winsberg, 1977), abdominal cramps, diarrhea, irritability, oppositional behavior, and withdrawal dyskinesia. Patients with Tourette's may have an exacerbation of symptoms during dosage reduction that may occur for several months. This phenomenon complicates decisions about the effectiveness of the medication and the need for further treatment (Cohen, Riddle, and Leckman, 1992).

SPECIAL INSTRUCTIONS FOR PARENTS/CARE GIVERS/ CHILDREN/ADOLESCENTS

- Anti-psychotics may cause drowsiness during the first few weeks of therapy. If this happens, the patient should not participate in activities that require alertness, such as riding a bike or driving a car.

- For patients taking chlorpromazine, thioridazine, mesoridazine, or pimozide an electrocardiogram will need to be done before starting the medication.
- For patients taking clozapine, a weekly blood test is necessary to watch for a decrease in white blood cells. Clozapine tablets will only be available through a special program designed to ensure a weekly blood test is done. Be sure to tell the physician if the patient develops any sign of infection (sore throat, sores in the mouth), fever, or becomes tired or weak.
- If the patient develops severe muscle stiffness, high fever, increased heart rate, or slow movements, stop the medication and contact the physician immediately.
- If the patient develops uncontrolled movements of any part of the body, yellow eyes or skin, skin rash, sore throat, infections, inability to urinate, mental confusion, irregular pulse, seizures, or any other unusual reaction, contact the physician as soon as possible.
- These medications will make the skin more sensitive to sunburn. Be sure to use a sunscreen lotion and wear protective clothing when outside. These medications also tend to allow the body to overheat; be sure to drink plenty of water and restrict your physical activity in hot weather. Avoid the use of hot tubs, saunas, or other hot environments while taking this medication.
- For a dry mouth, use sugarless gum or candy. You may also rinse your mouth with water or suck on pieces of ice.
- Do not stop taking this medication abruptly. The physician will want to decrease the dose gradually before stopping completely.
- Be sure to tell all physicians, pharmacists, and dentists that this medication is being taken.
- Do not take any other medications without checking with your physician or pharmacist.
- Liquid antipsychotics may be diluted in fruit juice or water just prior to administration.
- Store this medication and all medication away from the patient and other children and adolescents.

• This medication should not be taken during pregnancy, due to the risks of birth defects.
• Avoid the use of alcoholic beverages during therapy with this medication.

PRODUCTS AVAILABLE

Chlorpromazine is available as Thorazine® from SmithKline French. Thorazine® is marketed in non-scored orange tablets, liquids, and injectable form. Thorazine® 10 mg is imprinted with SKF T 73. Thorazine® 25 mg is imprinted with SKF T 74. Thorazine® 50 mg is imprinted with SKF T 76. Thorazine® 100 mg is imprinted with SKF T 77. Thorazine® 200 mg is imprinted with SKF T 79. There are two Thorazine® concentrates that are custard flavored, and contain either chlorpromazine 30 mg per 1 ml or chlorpromazine 100 mg per 1 ml. Generic chlorpromazine products are available in the same dosage strengths.

Clozapine is available as Clozaril® from Sandoz Pharmaceuticals. Both Clozaril® tablets are pale yellow, round compressed tablets. Clozaril® 25 mg is imprinted with Clozaril 25. Clozaril® 100 mg is imprinted with Clozaril 100. Participation in the Clozaril® Patient Management System is required.

Fluphenazine hydrochloride is available as Permitil® from Schering and as Prolixon® from Bristol-Myers Squibb. Permitil® 2.5 mg is a light orange, oval, scored tablet imprinted with WDR 442. Permitil® 5 mg is purple-pink, oval, scored tablet imprinted with WFF 550. Permitil® 10 mg is a light red, oval, scored tablet imprinted with WFF 550. Permitil® concentrate contains fluphenazine 5 mg per 1 ml and is unflavored. Prolixin® 1.0 mg is a pink tablet. Prolixin® 2.5 mg is a yellow tablet. Prolixin® 5 mg is a green tablet. Prolixin-® 10 mg is a coral tablet. All of the Prolixin® tablets contain tartrazine. Prolixin® elixir contains fluphenazine 2.5 mg per 5 ml and is orange flavored. Prolixin® concentrate contains fluphenazine 5 mg per 1 ml. Fluphenazine is also available in generic form.

Haloperidol is available as Haldol® from McNeil Pharmaceuticals. All of the Haldol® tablets are scored, horseshoe shaped, with an H cut out in the center and imprinted with Haldol/McNeil. Haldol® 0.5 mg is white and imprinted with 1/2. Haldol® 1.0 mg is yellow and imprinted with a 1. Haldol® 2.0 mg is pink and imprinted with a 2. Haldol® 5 mg is green and imprinted with a 5. Haldol® 10 mg is aqua and is imprinted with a 10. Haldol® 20 mg is salmon colored and imprinted with a 20. Haldol® concentrate contains haloperidol 2 mg per 1 ml and is unflavored. Haloperidol is also available in generic form.

Loxapine is available as Loxitane® from Lederle Laboratories. Loxitane® 5 mg is a green capsule imprinted with L1 5 mg. Loxitane® 10 mg is a green and yellow capsule imprinted with L2 10 mg. Loxitane® 25 mg is a two-tone green capsule imprinted with L3 25 mg. Loxitane® 50 mg is a green and blue capsule imprinted with L4 50 mg. Loxitane C® contain loxapine 25 mg per 1 ml. Loxapine tablets are also available in generic form.

Mesoridazine is available as Serentil® from Boehringer Ingelheim. Serentil® is available in 10, 25, 50, and 100 mg tablets. Serentil® concentrate contains 25 mg per 1 ml.

Molindone is available as Moban® from DuPont Pharmaceuticals. All Moban® tablets are imprinted with DuPont/ Moban. Moban® 5 mg is an orange tablet imprinted with a 5. Moban® 10 mg is a lavender tablet imprinted with a 10. Moban® 25 mg is a light green tablet imprinted with a 25. Moban® 50 mg is a blue tablet imprinted with a 50. Moban® 100 mg is a tan tablet imprinted with a 100. Moban® concentrate contains molindone 20 mg per 1 ml and is cherry flavored.

Pimozide is available as Orap® from Lemmon Pharmaceuticals. Orap® 2 mg is a white, oval, scored tablet imprinted with Orap 2.

Thioridazine is available as Mellaril® from Sandoz Pharmaceuticals. Mellaril® 10 mg is a bright chartreuse tablet imprinted with 78/2 S. Mellaril® 15 mg is a pink tablet imprinted with 78/8 S, 78/8 15 mg. Mellaril® 25 mg is a tan tablet imprinted with Mellaril 25 S, 78/3 25 mg. Mellaril® 50 mg is a white tablet imprinted with Mellaril S, 78/4, 50 mg. Mellaril® 100 mg is a green tablet imprinted with Mellaril 100 S, 78/5, 100 mg. Mellaril® 150 mg is a yellow tablet imprinted with Mellaril 150 S, 78/6, 150 mg. Mellaril® 200 mg is a pink tablet imprinted with Mellaril 200 S, 78/7, 200 mg. There are two Mellaril® concentrates that contain either thioridazine 30 mg per 1 ml or thioridazine 100 mg per 1 ml. There are two Mellaril suspensions that contain either thioridazine 25 mg per 5 ml or thioridazine 100 mg per 5 ml. Thioridazine is also available in generic form.

Thiothixene is available as Navane® from Roerig Pharmaceuticals. All Navane capsules are imprinted with Navane, Roerig. Navane® 1 mg is an orange and yellow capsule imprinted with 571. Navane® 2 mg is a yellow and light blue capsule imprinted with 572. Navane® 5 mg is an orange and white capsule imprinted with 573. Navane® 10 mg is a blue and white capsule imprinted with 574. Navane® 20 mg is a blue and light green capsule imprinted with 577. Navane® concentrate contains 5 mg per 1 ml and is fruit flavored. Thiothixene is also available in generic form.

COST

GENERIC NAME	TRADENAME	AWP*	AWP* per dose
Chlorpromazine 10 mg		$4.12 for 100 tablets	$0.05 per tablet
Chlorpromazine 25 mg		$4.71 for 100 tablets	$0.05 per tablet
Chlorpromazine 50 mg		$6.11 for 100 tablets	$0.07 per tablet
Chlorpromazine 100 mg		$7.07 for 100 tablets	$0.08 per tablet
Chlorpromazine 200 mg		$12.63 for 100 tablets	$0.13 per tablet
Chlorpromazine 30 mg per 1 ml concentrate		$6.65 for 100 ml	$0.07 per 1 ml
Chlorpromazine 100 mg per 1 ml concentrate		$8.22 for 100 ml	$0.09 per 1 ml

Chlorpromazine	Thorazine® 10 mg	$33.45 for 100 tablets	$0.34 per tablet
	Thorazine® 25 mg	$42.25 for 100 tablets	$0.43 per tablet
	Thorazine® 50 mg	$56.50 for 100 tablets	$0.57 per tablet
	Thorazine® 100 mg	$72.90 for 100 tablets	$0.73 per tablet
	Thorazine® (10 mg per 5 ml syrup)	$82.29 for 500 ml	$0.83 per 5 ml
	Thorazine® (30 mg per 1 ml concentrate)	$24.37 for 100 ml	$0.25 per 1 ml
	Thorazine® (100 mg per 1 ml concentrate)	$65.88 for 100 ml	$0.66 per 1 ml
Clozapine	Clozaril® 25 mg	$132.00 for 100 tablets	$1.32 per tablet
	Clozaril® 100 mg	$342.00 for 100 tablets	$3.42 per tablet
Fluphenazine 1 mg		$26.93 for 100 tablets	$0.27 per tablet
Fluphenazine 2.5 mg		$40.88 for 100 tablets	$0.41 per tablet
Fluphenazine 5 mg		$52.13 for 100 tablets	$0.53 per tablet
Fluphenazine 10 mg		$70.43 for 100 tablets	$0.71 per tablet
Fluphenazine	Prolixin® 1 mg	$76.74 for 100 tablets	$0.77 per tablet
	Prolixin® 2.5 mg	$108.68 for 100 tablets	$1.09 per tablet
	Prolixin® 5 mg	$140.20 for 100 tablets	$1.40 per tablet
	Prolixin® 10 mg	$182.67 for 100 tablets	$1.83 per tablet
	Prolixin® (2.5 mg per 5 ml elixir)	$140.62 for 500 ml	$1.41 per 5 ml
	Prolixin® (5 mg per 1 ml concentrate)	$87.47 for 100 ml	$0.88 per 1 ml
Fluphenazine	Permitil® 2.5 mg	$92.08 for 100 tablets	$0.93 per tablet
	Permitil® 5 mg	$122.92 for 100 tablets	$1.23 per tablet
	Permitil® 10 mg	$145.85 for 100 tablets	$1.46 per tablet
	Permitil® (5 mg per 1 ml concentrate)	$55.78 for 100 ml	$0.56 per 1 ml
Haloperidol 0.5 mg		$2.03 for 100 tablets	$0.03 per tablet
Haloperidol 1 mg		$2.10 for 100 tablets	$0.03 per tablet
Haloperidol 2 mg		$2.46 for 100 tablets	$0.03 per tablet
Haloperidol 5 mg		$2.76 for 100 tablets	$0.03 per tablet
Haloperidol 10 mg		$3.83 for 100 tablets	$0.04 per tablet
Haloperidol 20 mg		$11.85 for 100 tablets	$0.12 per tablet
Haloperidol concentrate 2 mg per 1 ml		$27.25 for 100 ml	$0.12 per 1 ml
Haloperidol	Haldol® 0.5 mg	$39.31 for 100 tablets	$0.40 per tablet
	Haldol® 1 mg	$58.19 for 100 tablets	$0.59 per tablet
	Haldol® 2 mg	$80.16 for 100 tablets	$0.81 per tablet
	Haldol® 5 mg	$131.17 for 100 tablets	$1.32 per tablet

	Haldol® 10 mg	$168.29 for 100 tablets	$1.69 per tablet
	Haldol® 20 mg	$322.85 for 100 tablets	$3.23 per tablet
	Haldol® (2 mg per 1 ml concentrate)	$76.44 for 100 ml	$0.77 per 1 ml
Loxapine 5 mg		$40.58 for 100 capsules	$0.41 per capsule
Loxapine 10 mg		$55.43 for 100 capsules	$0.56 per capsule
Loxapine 25 mg		$85.43 for 100 capsules	$0.86 per capsule
Loxapine 50 mg		$112.88 for 100 capsules	$1.13 per capsule
Loxapine	Loxitane® 5 mg	$79.07 for 100 capsules	$0.80 per capsule
	Loxitane® 10 mg	$102.17 for 100 capsules	$1.03 per capsule
	Loxitane® 25 mg	$154.39 for 100 capsules	$1.55 per capsule
	Loxitane® 50 mg	$205.98 for 100 capsules	$2.06 per capsule
	Loxitane C® (25 mg per 1 ml concentrate)	$189.57 for 100 ml	$1.90 per 1 ml
Mesoridazine	Serentil® 10 mg	$51.32 for 100 tablets	$0.52 per tablet
	Serentil® 25 mg	$68.69 for 100 tablets	$0.69 per tablet
	Serentil® 50 mg	$77.56 for 100 tablets	$0.78 per tablet
	Serentil® 100 mg	$94.80 for 100 tablets	$0.95 per tablet
	Serentil® (25 mg per 1 ml concentrate)	$37.48 for 100 ml	$0.38 per 1 ml
Molindone	Moban® 5 mg	$51.88 for 100 tablets	$0.52 per tablet
	Moban® 10 mg	$74.53 for 100 tablets	$0.75 per tablet
	Moban® 25 mg	$111.17 for 100 tablets	$1.12 per tablet
	Moban® 50 mg	$148.46 for 100 tablets	$1.49 per tablet
	Moban® 100 mg	$198.33 for 100 tablets	$1.99 per tablet
	Moban® (20 mg per 1 ml concentrate)	$91.74 for 100 ml	$0.92 per 1 ml
Pimozide	Orap® 2 mg	$66.32 for 100 tablets	$0.67 per tablet
Thioridazine 10 mg		$3.69 for 100 tablets	$0.04 per tablet
Thioridazine 15 mg		$4.82 for 100 tablets	$0.05 per tablet
Thioridazine 25 mg		$5.00 for 100 tablets	$0.05 per tablet
Thioridazine 50 mg		$7.13 for 100 tablets	$0.08 per tablet
Thioridazine 100 mg		$10.43 for 100 tablets	$0.11 per tablet
Thioridazine 150 mg		$21.47 for 100 tablets	$0.22 per tablet
Thioridazine 200 mg		$24.23 for 100 tablets	$0.25 per tablet
Thioridazine 30 mg per 1 ml concentrate		$10.75 for 100 ml	$0.11 per 1 ml
Thioridazine 100 mg per 1 ml concentrate		$32.21 for 100 ml	$0.33 per 1 ml
Thioridazine	Mellaril® 10 mg	$26.88 for 100 tablets	$0.27 per tablet
	Mellaril® 15 mg	$31.68 for 100 tablets	$0.32 per tablet
	Mellaril® 25 mg	$37.80 for 100 tablets	$0.38 per tablet

Mellaril® 50 mg	$45.90 for 100 tablets	$0.46 per tablet
Mellaril® 100 mg	$55.92 for 100 tablets	$0.56 per tablet
Mellaril® 150 mg	$70.98 for 100 tablets	$0.71 per tablet
Mellaril® 200 mg	$80.88 for 100 tablets	$0.81 per tablet
Mellaril® (30 mg per 1 ml concentrate)	$24.20 for 100 ml	$0.25 per 1 ml
Mellaril® (100 mg per 1 ml concentrate)	$63.25 for 100 ml	$0.64 per 1 ml
Mellaril® (25 mg per 5 ml suspension)	$47.63 for 500 ml	$0.48 per 5 ml
Mellaril® (100 mg per 5 ml suspension)	$97.94 for 500 ml	$0.98 per 5 ml
Thiothixene 1 mg	$9.75 for 100 capsules	$0.10 per capsule
Thiothixene 2 mg	$12.75 for 100 capsules	$0.13 per capsule
Thiothixene 5 mg	$17.78 for 100 capsules	$0.18 per capsule
Thiothixene 10 mg	$26.63 for 100 capsules	$0.27 per capsule
Thiothixene 20 mg	$59.93 for 100 capsules	$0.60 per capsule
Thiothixene 5 mg per 1 ml concentrate	$21.56 for 100 ml	$0.22 per 1 ml
Thiothixene Navane® 1 mg	$36.56 for 100 capsules	$0.37 per capsule
Navane® 2 mg	$49.30 for 100 capsules	$0.50 per capsule
Navane® 5 mg	$77.09 for 100 capsules	$0.78 per capsule
Navane® 10 mg	$106.24 for 100 capsules	$1.07 per capsule
Navane® 20 mg	$163.91 for 100 capsules	$1.64 per capsule
Navane® (5 mg per 1 ml concentrate)	$65.54 for 100 ml	$0.66 per 1 ml

* AWP is the average wholesale price to the pharmacist that is listed in the *1994 Redbook* (Cardinale, 1994).

REFERENCES

Anderson, LT, Campbell, M, Grega, DM, Perry, R, Small, AM, Green, WH. Haloperidol in the treatment of infantile autism: Effects on learning and behavioral symptoms. *Am J Psych,* 1984;141:1195-1202.

Anderson, LT, Campbell, M, Adams, P, Small, AM, Perry, R, Shell, J. The effects of haloperidol on discrimination learning and behavioral symptoms in autistic children. *J Autism Dev Disorders,* 1989;19:227-239.

Apter, A, Dickermann, Z, Gonen, N, Assa, S, Prager-Lewin, R, Kaufman, H, Tyano, S, Laron, Z. Effect of chlorpromazine on hypothalamic-pituitary-gonadal function in 10 adolescent schizophrenic boys. *Am J Psych,* 1983;140:1588-1591.

Bennett, WG, Kalmijn, M, Grega, D, Campbell, M. Electroencephalogram and treatment of hospitalized aggressive children with haloperidol or lithium. *Biol Psych,* 1983;18:1427-1440.

Birmaher, B, Baker, R, Kapur, S, Quintana, H, Ganguli, R. Clozapine for the treatment of adolescents with schizophrenia. *J Amer Acad Child Adolesc Psychiatry,* 1992;31:160-164.

Blanz, B, Schmidt, MH. Clozapine for schizophrenia. *J Amer Acad Child Adolesc Psychiatry,* 1993;32:223-224.

Bornstein, RA, Yang, V. Neuropsychological performance in medicated and unmedicated patients with Tourette's disorder. *Am J Psych,* 1991;148:468-471.

Boxer, G, Davidson, J. More on clozapine. *J Amer Acad Child Adolesc Psychiatry,* 1992;31:993.

Bruun, RD. Gilles de la Tourette's syndrome: An overview of clinical experience. *J Amer Acad Child Psychiatry,* 1984;23:126-133.

Bruun, RD. Subtle and underrecognized side effects of neuroleptic treatment in children with Tourette's disorder. *Am J Psych,* 1988;145:621-624.

Campbell, M, Anderson, LT, Meier, M, Cohen, IL, Small, AM, Samit, C, Sacher, ES. A comparison of haloperidol and behavior therapy and their interaction in autistic children. *J Amer Acad Child Psychiatry,* 1978;17:640-655.

Campbell, M. On the use of neuroleptics in children and adolescents. *Psych Annals,* 1985;15:101-107.

Campbell, M, Cohen, IL, Small, AM. Drugs in aggressive behavior. *J Amer Acad Child Psychiatry,* 1982;21:107-117.

Campbell, M, Grega, DM, Green, WH, Bennett, WG. Neuroleptic-induced dyskinesias in children. *Clin Neuropharmacol,* 1983;6:207-222.

Campbell, M, Adams, P, Perry, R, Spencer, EK, Overall, JE. Tardive and withdrawal dyskinesia in autistic children: A prospective study. *Psychopharm Bull,* 1988;24:251-255.

Campbell, M, Small, AM, Green, WH, Jennings, SJ, Perry, R, Bennett, WG, Anderson, L. Behavioral efficacy of haloperidol and lithium carbonate. *Arch Gen Psych,* 1984;41:650-656.

Cardinale, VA (ed). *1994 Drug Topics Redbook,* Medical Economic Company, Inc., 1994; 139, 148, 198, 208, 209, 258, 264, 289, 314, 322, 340, 361, 383, 385.

Chandler, JD. Propranolol treatment of akathesia in Tourette's syndrome. *J Amer Acad Child Adolesc Psychiatry,* 1990;29:475-477.

Cohen, DJ, Riddle, MA, Leckman, JF. Pharmacotherapy of Tourette's syndrome and associated disorders. *Pysch Clinic North Amer,* 1992;15:109-129.

Diamond, JM, Hayes, DD. A case of neuroleptic malignant syndrome in a mentally retarded adolescent. *J Adolesc Health Care,* 1986;7:419-422.

Ernst, M, Magee, HJ, Gonzalez, NM, Locascio, JJ, Rosenberb, CR, Campbell, M. Pimozide in autistic children. *Psychopharm Bull,* 1992;28:187-191.

Ernst, M, Gonzalez, NM, Campbell, M. Acute dystonic reaction with low-dose pimozide. *J Amer Acad Child Adolesc Psychiatry,* 1993;32:640-642.

Frazier, JA, Gordon, CT, McKenna, K, Lenane, M, Jih, D, Rapoport, JL. An open trial of clozapine in 11 adolescents with childhood-onset schizophrenia. *J Amer Acad Child Adolesc Psychiatry,* 1994;33:658-663.

Freedman, JE, Wirshing, WC, Russell, AT, Bray, MP, Unutzer J. Absence status seizures during successful long-term clozapine treatment of an adolescent with schizophrenia. *J Child Adolesc Psychopharmacology,* 1994;4:53-62.

Gonzalez, A, Michanie, C. Clozapine for refractory psychosis. *J Amer Acad Child Adolesc Psychiatry,* 1992;31:1169-1170.

Grob, CS. Persistent supersensitivity vomiting following neuroleptic withdrawal in an adolescent. *Biol Psych,* 1986;21:398-401.

Gualtieri, CT, Patterson, DR. Neuroleptic-induced tics in two hyperactive children. *Am J Psych,* 1986;143:1176-1177.

Jacobsen, LK, Walker, MC, Edwards, JE, Chappell, PB, Woolston, JL. Clozapine in the treatment of a young adolescent with schizophrenia. *J Amer Acad Child Adolesc Psychiatry,* 1994;33:645-650.

Joshi, PT, Capozzoli, JA, Coyle, JT. Low-dose neuroleptic therapy for children with childhood-onset pervasive developmental disorder. *Am J Psych,* 1988; 145:335-338.

Joshi, PT, Capozzoli, J, Coyle, J. Neuroleptic malignant syndrome: Life threatening complication of neuroleptic treatment in adolescents with affective disorders. *Pediatrics,* 1991;87:235-239.

Karagianis, JL, Nagpurkar, R. A case of Tourette syndrome developing during haloperidol treatment. *Can J Psych,* 1990;35:228-232.

Keepers, GA, Clappison, VJ, Casey, DE. Initial anticholinergic prophylaxis for neuroleptic-induced extrapyramidal syndromes. *Arch Gen Psych,* 1983;40: 1113-1117.

Kutcher, S, Williamson, P, MacKenzie, S, Marton, P, Ehrlich, M. Successful clonazepam treatment of neuroleptic-induced akathisa in older adolescents and young adults: A double-blind, placebo-controlled study. *J Clin Psychopharmacol,* 1989;9:403-406.

Kutcher, SP, Mackenzie, S, Galarraga, W, Szalai, J. Clonazepam treatment of adolescents with neuroleptic-induced akathisia. *Am J Psych,* 1987;144: 823-824.

Latz, SR, McCracken, JT. Neuroleptic malignant syndrome in children and adolescents: Two case reports and a warning. *J Child Adolesc Psychopharmacology,* 1992;2:123-129.

Levkovitch, Y, Kaysar, N, Kronnenberg, Y, Hagai, H, Gaoni, B. Clozapine for schizophrenia. *J Amer Acad Child Adolesc Psychiatry,* 1994;33:431.

Linet, LS. Tourette syndrome, pimozide and school phobia: The neuroleptic separation anxiety syndrome. *Am J Psych,* 1985; 142: 613-615.

McClellan, JM, Werry, JS. Schizophrenia. *Psych Clinic North America,* 1992; 15:131-148.

Meiselas, KD, Spencer, EK, Oberfield, R, Peselow, ED, Angrist, B, Campbell, M. Differentiation of stereotypies from neuroleptic-related dyskinesias in autistic children. *J Clin Psychopharmacology,* 1989;9:207-209.

154   Psychiatric Drug Therapy for Children and Adolescents

Merry, SN, Werry, JS, Merry, AF, Birchall, N. The neuroleptic malignant syndrome in an adolescent. *J Amer Acad Child Psychiatry,* 1986;25:284-286.

Mikkelsen, EJ, Detlor, J, Cohen, DJ. School avoidance and social phobia triggered by haloperidol in patients with Tourette's disorder. *Am J Psych,* 1981;138:1572-1576.

Morselli, PL, Bianchetti, G, Dugas, M. Therapeutic drug monitoring of psychotropic drugs in children. *Pediat Pharmacol,* 1983;3:149-156.

Morselli, PL, Bianchetti, G, Durand, M, Heuzey, MF, Zarifian, E, Dugas, M. Haloperidol plasma level monitoring in pediatric patients. *Therap Drug Monitor,* 1979;1:35-46.

Mozes, T, Toren, P, Chernauzan, N, Mester, R, Yoran-Hegesh, R, Blumensohn, R, Wiseman, A. Clozapine treatment in very early onset schizophrenia. *J Amer Acad Child Adolesc Psychiatry,* 1994;33:65-70.

National Institutes of Mental Health. Abnormal Involuntary Movement Scale (AIMS). *Psychopharm Bull,* 1985;21:1077-1081.

Perry, R, Nobler, MS, Campbell, M. Tourette-like symptoms associated with neuroleptic therapy in an autistic child. *J Amer Acad Child Adolesc Psychiatry,* 1989;28:93-96.

Perry, R, Campbell, M, Adams, P, Lynch, N, Spencer, EK, Curren, EL, Overall, JE. Long-term efficacy of haloperidol in autistic children: Continuous versus discontinuous drug administration. *J Amer Acad Child Adolesc Psychiatry,* 1989;28:87-92.

Physician's Desk Reference. Oradell, NJ. Medical Economic Data, 1994.

Platt, JE, Campbell, M, Green, WH, Grega, DM. Cognitive effects of lithium carbonate and haloperidol in treatment resistant aggressive children. *Arch Gen Psych,* 1984;41:657-662.

Poole, D, Bloom, W, Mielke, DH, Roniger, JJ, Gallant, DM. A controlled evaluation of loxitane in seventy-five adolescent schizophrenic patients. *Curr Therap Res,* 1976;19:99-104.

Realmuto, GM, Erickson, WD, Yellin, AM, Hopwood, JH, Greenberg, LM. Clinical comparison of thiothixene and thioridazine in schizophrenic adolescents. *Am J Psych,* 1984;141:440-442.

Remschmidt, H, Schulz, E, Martin, PD. An open trial of clozapine in thirty-six adolescents with schizophrenia. *J Child Adolesc Psychopharmacology,* 1994;4:31-41.

Riddle, MA, Hardin, MT, Towbin, KE, Leckamn, JF, Cohen, DJ. Tardive dyskinesia following haloperidol treatment in Tourette's syndrome. *Arch Gen Psych,* 1987;44:98-99.

Salle, FR, Pollock, BG, Stiller, RL, Stull, S, Everett, G, Perel, JM. Pharmacokinetics of pimozide in adults and children with Tourette's syndrome. *J Clin Pharmacol,* 1987;27:776-781.

Shapiro, AK, Shapiro, E. Clinical efficacy of haloperidol, pimozide, penfluridol and clonidine in the treatment of Tourette syndrome. In *Advances in Neurology.* 1982. Vol. 35. Edited by Friedhoff, AJ and Chase, TN. New York: Raven Press.

Shapiro, AK, Shapiro, E. Controlled study of pimozide versus placebo in Tourette's syndrome. *J Amer Acad Child Psych,* 1984;23:161-173.

Shapiro, AK, Shapiro, E, Eisenkraft GJ. Treatment of Gilles de la Tourette syndrome with pimozide. *Am J Psych,* 1983;140:1183-1186.

Shapiro, E, Shapiro, AK, Fulop, G, Hubbard, M, Mandeli, J, Nordlie, J, Phillips, RA. Controlled study of haloperidol, pimozide, and placebo for the treatment of Gilles de la Tourette's syndrome. *Arch Gen Psych,* 1989;46:722-730.

Silva, RR, Magee, HJ, Friedhoff, AJ. Persistent tardive dyskinesia and other neuroleptic-related dyskinesias in Tourette's disorder. *J Child Adolesc Psychopharmacology,* 1993a;3:137-144.

Silva, RR, Malone, RP, Anderson, LT, Shay, J, Campbell, M. Haloperidol withdrawal and weight changes in autistic children. *Psychopharm Bull,* 1993b; 29:287-291.

Singer, HS, Gammon, K, Quaskey, S. Haloperidol, fluphenazine and clonidine in Tourette syndrome: Controversies in treatment. *Pediat Neurosci,* 1985-86; 12:71-74.

Spencer, EK, Kafantaris, V, Padron-Gayol, MV, Rosenberg, CR, Campbell, M. Haloperidol in schizophrenic children: Early findings from a study in progress. *Psychopharm Bull,* 1992;28:183-186.

Sprague, RL, Kalachnik, JE. Reliability, validity and a total score cutoff for the Dyskinesia Identification System: Condensed User Scale (DISCUS) with mentally ill and mentally retarded populations. *Psychopharm Bull,* 1991;27:51-58.

Sramek, JJ, Simpson, GM, Morrison, RL, Heiser, JF. Anticholinergic agents for prophylaxis of neuroleptic-induced dystonic reactions: A prospective study. *J Clin Psych,* 1986;47:305-309.

Steingard, R, Khan, A, Gonzalez, A, Herzog, DB. Neuroleptic malignant syndrome: Review of experience with children and adolescents. *J Child Adolesc Psychopharmacology,* 1992;2:183-198.

Sylvester, C. Psychopharmacology of disorders in children. *Psych Clinic North Amer,* 1993;16:779-791.

Teicher, MH, Glod, CA. Neuroleptic drugs: Indications and guidelines for their rational use in children and adolescents. *J Child Adolesc Psychopharmacol,* 1990;1:33-56.

Tenenbein, M. The neuroleptic malignant syndrome: Occurrence in a 15-year-old boy and recovery with bromocriptine therapy. *Ped Neurosci,* 1985/86; 12:161-164.

Towbin, KE, Dykens, EM, Pugliese, RG. Clozapine for early developmental delays with childhood-onset of schizophrenia: Protocol and 15-month outcome. *J Amer Acad Child Adolesc Psychiatry,* 1994;33:651-657.

United States Pharmacopeia, Drug Information, 1994, Volumes I and II. Sections on antipsychotics.

Weiden, P, Bruun, R. Worsening of Tourette's disorder due to neuroleptic-induced akathisa. *Am J Psych,* 1987;144:504-505.

Whitaker, A, Rao, U. Neuroleptics in pediatric psychiatry. *Psych Clinic North Amer,* 1992;15:243-276.

Woodbury, MM, Woodbury, MA. Neuroleptic-induced catatonia as a stage in the progression toward neuroleptic malignant syndrome. *J Amer Acad Child Adolesc Psychiatry,* 1992;31:1161-1164.

Yepes, LE, Winsberg, BG. Vomiting during neuroleptic withdrawal in children. *Am J Psych,* 1977;134:574.

Chapter 4

Lithium

Lithium carbonate

> Eskalith® and Eskalith CR® are marketed by SmithKline Beecham.
>
> Lithonate® and Lithotab® are marketed by Solvay.
>
> Lithane® is marketed by Miles Pharmaceuticals.
>
> Lithium carbonate is available in generic form.

Lithium citrate syrup

> Lithium citrate is available in generic form.

DSM-IV INDICATIONS

Bipolar disorder in adolescents

Bipolar disorder in prepubertal children (??)

Conduct disorder, with aggression (???)

> FDA: Not indicated for children less than 12 years old (*PDR*, 1994).
> USP: Appropriate studies on the relationship of age to the effects of lithium have not been performed in the pediatric population (*USPDI*, 1994).

CONTRAINDICATIONS: Pregnancy; breast-feeding; renal, thyroid, and cardiovascular disease or dysfunction; dehydration or susceptibility to dehydration; severe acne, psoriasis; hyponatremia, hypokalemia; disorders of bone formation or density; leukemia or history of leukemia; hypothyroidism; hyperparathyroidism; urinary retention; low sodium diets; low intake of water or fluids; and for the Lithane® product, tartrazine sensitivity.

PHARMACOLOGY: Lithium has numerous pharmacological effects on the central nervous system ion channels, neurotransmitters, and second-messenger systems. Second-messenger systems include the phosphoinositides (PI) and cyclic AMP (Alessi et al., 1994). Lithium down-regulates some serotonergic receptor subtypes and increases serotonin turnover. This results in a reduction of negative feedback, thereby increasing the release of serotonin. Lithium treatment has been reported to decrease total beta-receptor binding and to increase the release of norepinephrine. Lithium also increases dopamine levels and turnover and blocks the up-regulation of dopamine receptors when given concurrently with neuroleptics (Alessi et al., 1994). The exact mechanism of action of lithium in the treatment of bipolar disorder and depression is unknown.

Lithium, as a monovalent cation, competes with other monovalent and divalent cations (sodium, potassium, magnesium, calcium) at cell membranes, cellular binding sites, and cellular proteins. By replacing these ions intracellularly, lithium can alter the properties of excitable neurons, interfere with neurosecretory processes and membrane transport, and block enzyme activation. By inhibiting adenylate cyclase, lithium reduces intracellular concentrations of cyclic AMP. By inhibiting vasopressin-stimulated adenylate cyclase, lithium induces nephrogenic diabetes insipidus. Lithium also inhibits the activity of adenylate cyclase in the thyroid, resulting in a decreased release of thyroxine and triiodothyronine. In addition, lithium inhibits the synthesis and release of testosterone. The studies of lithium's effect on bone composition and metabolism in animals and adults have produced conflicting results (Jefferson et al., 1987). There are no studies of bone development in children and adolescents who are taking lithium. Lithium has diverse biochemical and physiological effects. The implications of the effect of lithium on growth and maturation in children and adolescents are unknown (Jefferson et al., 1987).

STUDIES OF LITHIUM EFFICACY

Bipolar Disorder

Varanka et al. (1988) reported an open study of the effects of lithium therapy in ten children (aged six to 12 years) with psychotic symptoms during mania. Each of the children received doses of lithium between 1,150 and 1,800 mg/day. Lithium levels were between 0.6 and 1.4 mEq/L and were obtained within three to five days after initiation of lithium therapy. Improvement was noted within an average of 11 days (range three to 24 days) after beginning lithium therapy.

DeLong and Nieman (1983) reported the effects of lithium in 16 outpatients (ages 6.3 to 13.5 years) with symptoms suggestive of mania. The patients suffered onset of difficulties between the ages two and nine years. Eleven of the 16 subjects participated in a double-blind, placebo-controlled, crossover study of lithium. Parents rated the children as significantly better on lithium. Lithium administration was associated with a significant improvement in explosive violent outbursts, aggressive behavior, mood swings, and both manic and depressive extremes of mood. In a clinical report, Delong and Aldershof (1987) reported the long-term efficacy of lithium therapy in childhood behavior disorders by diagnosis. In this report, lithium therapy was most useful for children with bipolar disorder, emotionally unstable character disorder, and for offspring of a lithium-responsive parent. Lithium was not effective for children with ADHD.

Strober et al. (1990) reported an 18-month naturalistic study of relapse following discontinuation of lithium maintenance therapy in 37 adolescents, 13 to 17 years of age. Each patient was diagnosed with mania with no psychotic features. Thirteen of the patients discontinued prophylactic lithium therapy shortly after discharge from the hospital. The relapse rate of these patients (92.3 percent) was nearly three times higher than the rate in patients who continued lithium prophylaxis therapy (37.5 percent). Patients who continued lithium therapy had a decreased frequency of affective illnesses while receiving lithium compared to baseline. This report suggests that lithium carbonate is an effective prophylactic agent that may prevent or decrease relapses for adolescents with bipolar disorder.

Aggression

Campbell et al. (1984) conducted a double-blind, placebo-controlled study of 61 hospitalized children (aged 5.2 to 12.9 years) with aggressive and explosive conduct disorder. These children did not have affective symptoms or a family history of affective illness. The study compared the effects of haloperidol and lithium, and both drugs were found to be significantly superior to placebo. Lithium doses ranged from 500 to 2,000 mg/day with a mean of 1,166 mg/day. Lithium serum concentrations ranged from 0.32 to 1.51 mEq/L with a mean of 0.993 mEq/L. Haloperidol doses varied from 1 to 6 mg/day with a mean of 2.95 mg/day. The target symptoms in this study were severe aggressiveness, explosiveness, and disruptiveness that were unresponsive to various outpatient treatments including pharmacotherapy. In this study, haloperidol was associated with more adverse effects than lithium. The lithium adverse effects included weight gain, stomachache, headache, fatigue, and tremor. None of the patients had a seizure disorder, however, 58 percent of the patients had a variety of electroencephalographic abnormalities. There were no reports of seizures while taking lithium (Campbell et al., 1984). The drug effects on cognition were considered mild, but the cognitive effects of lithium were less than with haloperidol (Platt et al., 1984).

Campbell, Gonzalez, and Silva (1992) indicate that no single treatment of aggression yields dramatic and long-lasting results. In addition, aggression is a low frequency behavior and is difficult to monitor and assess. A two-week baseline assessment should be utilized to observe target behaviors before drug therapy is indicated. Lithium is most beneficial for children with aggressive and destructive behaviors that are accompanied by explosiveness. Children with aggressive behaviors need psychosocial therapy as well as pharmacotherapy. Pharmacotherapy cannot be expected to resolve adverse family and environmental influences including a chaotic household and parental psychopathology (Campbell, Gonzalez, and Silva, 1992).

There is suggestive data from open trials that mentally retarded patients with aggression and explosiveness have a good response to lithium (Dale, 1980; Dostal and Zvolsky, 1970). The polyuria and polydipsia that results from lithium therapy can be a serious management problem. It is an interesting observation that for one patient reported by Dale (1980) enuresis ceased with lithium therapy. This is in contrast to the observation that lithium may induce enuresis (Dostal and Zvolsky, 1970). These findings warrant a double-blind, placebo-controlled trial to more fully determine the effectiveness of lithium in aggressive mentally retarded persons.

Depression

There are two reported open trials of lithium augmentation of tricyclic antidepressants in adolescents (Strober et al., 1992; Ryan et al., 1988). Ryan et al. (1988) conducted a retrospective chart review of 14 depressed adolescents who were treated with a tricyclic antidepressant for at least six weeks followed by the addition of lithium. Six of the 14 patients were rated as responders to lithium augmentation. The responders experienced a gradual improvement in symptoms over the first month of lithium therapy. The authors acknowledge that some patients may have improved with time, due of the fluctuating nature of the illness. Because of the lack of response to the tricyclic antidepressant it is also possible that only the lithium was effective. Strober et al. (1992) conducted a three-week open trial of lithium augmentation in 24 adolescents who remained highly depressed after six weeks of imipramine therapy. Two patients had a dramatic response within the first week and an additional eight patients showed a partial improvement. These preliminary reports suggest that lithium may be helpful in a limited number of patients with treatment resistant depression.

DEVELOPMENTAL PHARMACOKINETICS

Absorption: Lithium from regular release formulation is rapidly absorbed. Vitiello et al. (1988) reported a mean peak serum concentration, from nine children, of 2.4 hours with a range of one to four hours. Controlled release lithium has not been investigated in children.

Onset of action: Depending upon the diagnosis, lithium effects can be seen within two days to six weeks.

Duration of action: The duration of action is variable and has not been studied. Most children require a two or three times a day dosing regimen.

Half-life: In a study of nine children with conduct disorder, aged nine to 12 years, the half-life ranged from 10.4 to 34.6 hours with a mean of 17.9 hours (Vitiello et al., 1988). The reported mean half-life of 17.9 hours from this study is shorter than the reported mean half-life of 21 hours in adults. The wide variation in half-lives for these nine children suggests further investigations are needed. There are no pharmacokinetic studies in adolescents (Alessi et al., 1994).

Serum levels/saliva levels: A therapeutic serum level in children has not been investigated. Most studies use the range of 0.6 to 1.2 mEq/L. Therapeutic serum lithium levels in adults are in the range of 0.6 to 1.2 mEq/L, however, recent reports suggest that some adults respond to lithium levels of 0.3 to 0.6 mEq/L (Shader and Greenblatt, 1992; Himmelhoch, 1994). It is possible that some children and adolescents will respond to lower lithium serum levels as well. The ratio of saliva to serum lithium levels varies per individual. In order to monitor saliva lithium levels, several simultaneous saliva and serum lithium levels need to be drawn in order to determine the saliva-serum ratio for a particular patient. Saliva levels are currently not routinely recommended (Vitiello et al., 1988; Alessi et al., 1994).

DOSAGE RANGES

Lithium carbonate 300 mg tablets or capsules contain 8 mEq of lithium. Lithium citrate syrup contains 8 mEq of lithium per 5 ml. Lithium serum levels are proportional to the dose administered. Increases or decreases in dose will result in a proportional increase or decrease in serum levels (Fetner and Geller, 1992).

For adolescents: In the treatment of acute mania, lithium doses, for the regular release formulations and for the syrup, are initiated at 300 to 600 mg three times daily. Dosage adjustments are based on response and according to lithium serum levels. For the extended release formulations of lithium, initial doses are 450 to 900 mg two times daily with subsequent dosage adjustments.

For children up to the age of 12 years: Lithium doses, for the regular release formulations and for the syrup are initiated at 15 to 20 mg per kg of body weight administered in two to three divided doses. Due to the wide variability in half-life of lithium in children (Vitiello et al., 1988), it is recommended that lithium be administered in divided doses in order to maintain more constant blood levels. There is a wide range of resultant lithium serum levels per dose administered (Vitiello et al., 1988). Dosage has not been established for the extended release formulations of lithium for children.

DOSAGE PREDICTIONS

Dosage predictions of lithium are utilized to obtain a therapeutic lithium blood level in a shorter period of time and to decrease the number of blood drawings. Obtaining a therapeutic lithium blood level more quickly may or may not result in a faster onset of therapeutic action. Dosage predictions may be helpful as a guide to ultimate lithium dose. Two preliminary investigations have been conducted to determine the usefulness of lithium dosage predictions.

Weller, Weller, and Fristad (1986) conducted an investigation in 15 hospitalized prepubertal children, aged six to 12 years, on the use of a lithium dosage schedule. Initial lithium doses were based on the weight of the patient (30 mg/kg/day) and were administered in three divided doses with meals. The weights of the patients varied from 21.2 to 47.0 kg with corresponding lithium dosages of 600 to 1,200 mg/day. Lithium levels were drawn in the morning on days two, four, and six. On day two, nine out of 15 lithium serum levels were reported and varied from 0.5 to 0.9 mEq/L. On day four, 14 out of 15 lithium serum levels were reported and varied from 0.4

to 1.5 mEq/L, and on day six, 11 out of 15 lithium serum levels were reported and varied from 0.6 to 1.7 mEq/L. The clinical response of the patients was not reported, but the authors indicate that most patients showed improvement. Two of the 15 patients had lithium serum levels beyond the range of 1.2 mEq/L. This preliminary investigation requires replication, but suggests that the excretion of lithium is variable in children, and using a lithium dose based on the weight of the child results in a wide variation in serum lithium levels.

Geller and Fetner (1989) used the Cooper nomogram of dose predictions in six children (Cooper, Bergner, and Simpson, 1973). The test requires the administration of a 600 mg dose of lithium, followed by obtaining a serum lithium level at 24 hours. The Cooper nomogram correlates the 24-hour serum level and predicts the lithium dosage required to obtain a serum level of 0.6 to 1.2 mEq/L. The 24-hour serum lithium levels in this study were 0.3 mEq/L for each patient. This level is correlated with a lithium dose of 600 mg per day. The dosage predictions were accurate in two of the six subjects, but four subjects required increases in dosage from 300 to 600 mg/day. None of the subjects had excessive levels (Geller and Fetner, 1989).

The Cooper nomogram requires lithium serum level determinations down to 0.05 mEq/L. Clinical laboratories may or may not report lithium levels down to this level. Both of the lithium dosage prediction investigations described above used the lithium therapeutic range of 0.6 to 1.2 mEq/L. This lithium therapeutic range is currently under scrutiny for adult patients and it is suggested that some adults respond to lower lithium levels of 0.3 to 0.6 mEq/L (Shader and Greenblatt, 1992; Himmelhoch, 1994). It is possible that some children and adolescents will respond to lower lithium serum levels as well. In addition, the methods utilized in the above investigations resulted in varying lithium serum levels for the group of patients. Further investigations are needed to determine the utility of lithium dosage predictions in children. Each patient should be monitored individually and the lowest effective lithium dose should be administered.

ADVERSE EFFECTS REPORTED IN CHILDREN AND ADOLESCENTS

COMMON

Alessi et al. (1994) report that lithium therapy in children and adolescents is well tolerated. Side effects are infrequent and generally mild in short-term studies. It has been suggested that the frequency and severity of lithium side effects are less in children than in adults (Alessi et al., 1994). A baseline assessment should include appetite, eating and sleeping patterns, weight, blood pressure, heart rate, bowel and bladder control and tremor (Silva et al., 1992). Campbell et al. (1991) report that younger children had significantly more side effects in comparison to older children even when adjustments were made for weight, serum lithium levels, optimal dose, and duration of optimal dose. In addition, young autistic children had more frequent and more serious side effects than children of the same age diagnosed with conduct disorder. Predictors of lithium side effects appear to be age of the child and diagnosis. Patients with seizures, schizophrenia, and other neurological diseases may be more susceptible to lithium adverse effects even at subtherapeutic doses (Alessi et al., 1994). Teachers and other caretakers should be informed that the child is on lithium therapy, which requires extra water or fluid intake and may result in increased urination.

Weight gain: Lithium induced excessive weight gain may be due to fluid retention, the intake of high calorie drinks (polydipsia), hypothyroidism (see below), or a reduction in physical activity. Patients should be encouraged to maintain a normal diet and not restrict the amount of sodium chloride in their diet. The intake of water instead of high calorie fluids should also be encouraged. Weight loss has also been reported (Campbell et al., 1991) but does not appear to be as frequent as weight gain.

Diarrhea: Mild cases of diarrhea during the initial dosing period can be treated with lithium dosage reduction and maintaining sodium chloride in the diet. Moderate to severe diarrhea requires discontinuation of lithium. The controlled release formulation of lithium may be more likely to cause this effect.

Nausea: Administering lithium with food should reduce this side effect. If nausea occurs consistently, lithium serum levels should be checked.

Tremor: Dosage reduction is indicated. Restriction of caffeine intake is also advisable.

LESS COMMON

Metallic taste: Chewing sugarless gum or sucking on sugarless candy may alleviate this side effect.

Acne: Appropriate dermatological treatments are indicated. Tetracycline has been used to successfully treat lithium induced acne (Jefferson et al., 1987).

Skin rashes: Psoriasis may develop or be exacerbated. A maculopapular rash has also been reported in adults (Jefferson et al., 1987).

Nephrogenic diabetes insipidus: Polydipsia and polyuria, with a low urine specific gravity are signs of lithium induced diabetes insipidus. A reduction in the lithium dose is indicated.

Hypothyroidism: Signs and symptoms include depression, fatigue, intolerance to cold, edema, dry or rough hair, hair loss, elevation of thyroid stimulating hormone, and decreased T4 concentration. Hypothyroidism requires supplementation with levothyroxine (T4). Preliminary information suggests that this particular effect is uncommon in children (DeLong and Aldershof, 1987); however, there are several case reports of hypothyroidism (Alessi et al., 1994). Routine monitoring for hypothyroidism is indicated.

Growth: The effects of lithium on bone formation and density have not been studied in children. However, lithium may decrease bone formation or density in children by altering parathyroid hormone concentrations. Children with hypothyroidism are at increased risk of growth suppression. There are no case reports that suggest lithium causes growth impairment.

Hyperglycemia/Hypoglycemia: Lithium has a variable effect on blood glucose. Lithium is not contraindicated in diabetes mellitus, but closer monitoring of blood glucose is indicated (Jefferson et al., 1987).

Neutrophilia: An increase in white blood cells is frequently reported; however, the white blood cell count is usually within the normal range.

Enuresis: Dosage reduction or discontinuation is indicated. Therapy with a tricyclic antidepressant may be useful (Jefferson et al., 1987).

Nephrotoxicity: Long-term lithium administration and renal function have not been investigated in children or adolescents. Khandelwal, Varma, and Murthy (1984) reported on four adolescents (13 to 15 years old) who were given lithium for three to five years. Lithium levels were maintained between 0.5 and 1.0 mEq/L during this time period. None of the patients showed any glycosuria or proteinuria, or changes in serum creatinine, urine volume, or urine specific gravity. There are two separate reports of 14-year-old girls who developed proteinuria during a trial of lithium therapy. The proteinuria subsided after lithium discontinuation (Alessi et al., 1994).

Cardiac arrhythmia: Campbell et al. (1972) reported two five-year-old boys treated with lithium that developed reversible conduction defects. One boy developed a mild right ventricular conduction defect, and the other boy developed an atrioventricular nodal rhythm (*see also* Adverse Reactions/Case Reports). Cardiovascular effects in children appear to be rare and are infrequent in adults. Monitoring for fast or slow heartbeat, irregular pulse, and troubled breathing on exertion are suggested.

Teratogenic effect: Lithium is contraindicated during pregnancy, particularly during the first trimester. Lithium therapy during pregnancy is associated with an increased risk of congenital cardiovascular malformations (Jefferson et al., 1987).

ALLERGIC REACTION: Lithium preparations that contain tartrazine (e.g., Lithane®) may cause adverse reactions in sensitive individuals. Allergic reactions to lithium products are most likely due to the inactive ingredients of capsules and tablets. An allergic reaction to an element such as lithium is unlikely.

TOXICITY: Signs and symptoms of toxicity include confusion, word-finding difficulty, slurred speech, muscle twitching, weakness, lethargy, loss of appetite, nystagmus, ataxia, blurred vision, fever, hyperactive reflexes, seizures, cardiac arrhythmia, severe hypotension, tinnitus, obtundation, and coma. Toxicity in children may be more likely than in adults, due to dehydration associated with vomiting, diarrhea, fevers, infections, or aggressive dieting. Neurotoxicity may present even when lithium serum levels are in the "therapeutic range." Factors that predispose to lithium neurotoxicity are combination pharmacotherapy (lithium and neuroleptics), increasing age, seizure diathesis, schizophrenia, concurrent medical illness, and tissue retention of lithium (Alessi et al., 1994).

ADVERSE REACTIONS/CASE REPORTS

Cardiac Toxicity Associated with Lithium-Induced Hypothyroidism

Dietrich, Mortensen, and Wheller (1992) reported a 13-year-old male who developed hypothyroidism and severe congestive heart failure six months after he began taking lithium and imipramine for a severe conduct disorder. At the time of admission to the hospital the patient was taking 225 mg of imipramine and 2400 mg of lithium per day. The patient had no history of cardiac disease. Serum imipramine and desipramine levels were 176 ng/ml and serum lithium was 2.2 mEq/L. Thyroid indexes indicated decreased thyroxine and elevated thyroid stimulating hormone. Imipramine and lithium were discontinued and dobutamine, digoxin, furosemide, and spironolactone were initiated. One week after initiation of thyroid hormone replacement therapy, the patient developed potentially serious premature ventricular contractions. There was no ventricular tachycardia. Tocainide was initiated, and two days later the EKG was essentially normal. The patient was discharged on digoxin, furosemide, captopril, levothyroxine, and tocainide. The authors report that over the next 24 months, all medications but the tocainide and levothyroxine were discontinued. After three years, all medications were discontinued, and the patient remains difficult to manage due to the behavior disorder. The authors report that cardiac effects of lithium are infrequent and that the treated hypothyroidism may have contributed to this case. Monitoring for hypothyroidism is indicated for patients taking lithium, and the authors suggest the cardiac function be monitored for patients taking both lithium and a tricyclic antidepressant (Dietrich, Mortensen, and Wheller, 1992).

DRUG INTERACTIONS

DRUG	DRUGS	EFFECT
Lithium	Neuroleptics	May result in neurotoxicity with seizures, somnambulism, and an increased incidence of extrapyramidal symptoms. Neurotoxicity may occur at normal dosages and at therapeutic serum levels of lithium. Decreased phenothiazine blood levels and increased lithium concentration can occur. Chlorpromazine may increase the intracellular concentration of lithium. The mixing of lithium citrate syrup with neuroleptic liquids may result in the precipitation of the neuroleptic out of solution. Neuroleptics with anti-emetic effects may mask the early signs of lithium toxicity.
Lithium	Clozapine	Concurrent use will increase the risk of seizures, confusional states, neuroleptic malignant syndrome, and dyskinesias.

Lithium	Tricyclic antidepressants	The pharmacological effects of the tricyclic antidepressants may be increased (*see* Adverse Reactions/Case Reports).
Lithium	Non-steroidal anti-inflammatory	Lithium serum levels will be increased due to decreased renal clearance of lithium.
Lithium	Carbamazepine	Increased neurotoxic effects have been reported despite therapeutic blood levels of both drugs and normal doses. Lithium may reduce the anti-diuretic effects of carbamazepine and carbamazepine-induced leukopenia.
Lithium	Fluoxetine	Lithium serum levels can be increased by 40 percent; mechanism is unknown.
Lithium	Diuretics, loop and thiazide	Lithium serum levels will be increased. At least a 50 percent reduction of lithium dosage is necessary to avoid lithium toxicity.
Lithium	Calcium iodide, potassium iodide, iodinated glycerol, iodide salts, certain cough preparations	Lithium and other anti-thyroid drugs may potentiate the hypothyroid effects, if used concurrently.
Lithium	Neuromuscular blocking agents	Neuromuscular blocking effects may be increased; profound and severe respiratory depression may occur.
Lithium	Caffeine, aminophylline, dyphylline, oxtriphylline, theophylline	May result in increased lithium excretion excretion and decreased serum levels.
Lithium	Calcium channel blocking agents	Both increased and decreased lithium levels have occurred.
Lithium	Angiotensin-converting enzymes (ACE) inhibitors	Increases in lithium serum levels have been reported.

Lithium	Sodium bicarbonate, sodium chloride	High sodium intake can enhance lithium excretion.
Lithium	Metronidazole	Concurrent use may promote renal retention of lithium resulting in lithium toxicity.

MONITORING GUIDELINES

Baseline Assessment:

- History and physical, including weight, height, pulse, and blood pressure of the patient.
- White blood cell count (total and differential), serum electrolyte concentrations, serum calcium, serum phosphate, serum creatinine, thyroid function tests (serum thyroxine, thyroid stimulating hormone), urinalysis (urine specific gravity, urine proteins), serum beta-HCG pregnancy test in all females of child bearing potential, electrocardiogram if less than 16 or if cardiovascular disease is present. Optional: urine specific gravity after ten to 14-hour overnight fluid deprivation, electroencephalogram if neuromedical conditions are present.

Time Pattern for Response:

- For the treatment of aggression, it may take three to six weeks of lithium administration to achieve full therapeutic effectiveness (Campbell, Gonzalez, and Silva, 1992). For the treatment of mania, patients have responded within one to six weeks.

Follow-Up Assessment:

- Lithium serum levels should be obtained once per month (Fetner and Geller, 1992). Lithium serum levels are obtained ten to 12 hours after the last dose. Serum lithium levels are used as a guide to therapy (*see* Developmental Pharmacokinetics). Adverse effects may occur at low lithium serum levels. Check for signs and symptoms of hypothyroidism.

- Height and weight of the patient should be obtained every three months. Blood tests for renal function (blood urea nitrogen, serum creatinine, and urinalysis), thyroid function (thyroxine and thyroid stimulating hormone), serum calcium, serum phosphate, and electrolytes are recommended every three months or more often. For elevations of thyroid stimulating hormone, thyroxine supplementation is indicated. If urine specific gravity is less than 1.010 consider dose reduction. For hypoparathyroidism (hypercalcemia and hypophosphatemia) consider discontinuation of lithium.
- An electrocardiogram is indicated if cardiovascular adverse effects are present.
- Continue to educate the child and family regarding sodium chloride intake and dehydration effects.
- Duration of treatment is variable and according to the diagnosis.

Drug Discontinuation:

- Abrupt withdrawal may result in the return of the original symptoms. Sudden relapses have been reported with abrupt discontinuation; therefore, gradual withdrawal may be indicated.

SPECIAL INSTRUCTIONS FOR PARENTS/CARE GIVERS/CHILDREN/ADOLESCENTS

- Lithium should be taken with meals to avoid stomach upset.
- During lithium therapy, it is necessary to drink plenty of water, especially during hot weather or when exercising. The side effects of lithium increase if enough water is not consumed.
- It is important when taking lithium to maintain a steady amount of table salt (sodium chloride) in the diet. Avoid both large amounts of salt and especially very low amounts of salt in the diet. Changes in the diet should be done under the supervision of a physician.
- Lithium should be taken as prescribed by your physician. During the first few weeks of lithium therapy, blood tests are

done on a regular basis to determine the amount of lithium in your blood. After the dose is set, blood tests are done less often. Blood levels are usually drawn in the morning ten to 12 hours after the last dose of lithium. Lithium should not be taken the morning of the blood test. Take lithium after the blood test is done.

- Urine and other blood tests are also done to watch the effects of lithium.
- Common side effects of lithium are increased thirst and increased frequency of urination. Teachers should be informed that lithium therapy can result in an increased use of the bathroom and drinking fountain. Additional side effects are stomachache, nausea, diarrhea, vomiting, weight gain, fine hand tremor, tiredness, weakness, dizziness, and headache. If the patient develops an illness with vomiting, nausea, fever, dehydration, or loss of appetite, stop the lithium and call the physician. Lithium may decrease the activity of the thyroid gland. Patients with low thyroid activity may show signs of depression, continuing fatigue, dry or rough skin, hair loss, swelling of feet or lower legs, and sensitivity to cold. Other less common side effects of lithium are acne, skin rashes, hair loss, metallic taste, and bed wetting.
- Signs that lithium levels may be too high are vomiting or diarrhea more than once per day, severe hand tremor, weakness, lack of coordination, extreme sleepiness, severe dizziness, slurred speech, or trouble speaking. If these signs occur, stop the lithium and telephone the physician immediately.
- Signs of lithium toxicity are irregular heartbeat, fainting, confusion, staggering, blurred vision, ringing or buzzing in the ears, no urination, muscle twitches, high fever, convulsions, and unconsciousness.
- Common over-the-counter medications that should not be taken because the medications will increase lithium levels include ibuprofen (Advil®, Excedrin IB®, Medipren®, Midol 200®, Midol IB®, Motrin IB®, Nuprin®, Pamprin IB®, etc.); naproxen (Aleve®); and pamabrom, (Teen Midol®, Pamprin®, Midol PMS®). Before taking any other prescription or non-prescription medication, be sure to ask

the pharmacist or physician if it is okay to take the medication with lithium.
- Be sure to tell your pharmacist, dentist, and other physicians that you are taking lithium.
- Lithium therapy should be avoided during pregnancy due to the risk of birth defects.
- Store this medication and all medications away from the patient and other children and adolescents.

PRODUCTS AVAILABLE

Lithium carbonate and lithium citrate are available in several tradename and generic products listed below.
Lithium carbonate:

Eskalith® and Eskalith CR® are marketed by Smith-Kline Beecham. Eskalith® is available in both a capsule and tablet form. Eskalith® capsules have an opaque gray cap and an opaque yellow body, imprinted with the product name ESKALITH and SKF, and contain 300 mg of lithium carbonate. Eskalith® tablets are round, gray, scored, debossed with SKF and J09, and contain 300 mg of lithium carbonate. Eskalith CR® tablets are round, buff, scored, debossed with SKF J10, and contain 450 mg of lithium carbonate.

Lithonate® and Lithotab® are marketed by Solvay. Lithonate® capsules are peach colored, imprinted with Solvay 7512, and contain 300 mg of lithium carbonate. Lithotab® tablets are scored, white, film coated, imprinted with Solvay 7516, and contain 300 mg of lithium carbonate.

Lithane® is marketed by Miles Pharmaceuticals. Lithane® tablets are green, scored, imprinted with Miles 951, and contain 300 mg of lithium carbonate. Lithane® tablets also contain tartrazine.

Lithium carbonate is available in generic form as 150 mg and 300 mg capsules, and 300 mg tablets.

Lithium citrate syrup:
> Lithium citrate syrup is available in generic form and contains 8 mEq of lithium per 5 ml which is equivalent to 300 mg of lithium carbonate.

COST

GENERIC NAME	TRADENAME	AWP*	AWP* per dose
Lithium carbonate 150 mg		$7.63 for 100 capsules	$0.08 per capsule
Lithium carbonate 300 mg		$7.41 for 100 tablets	$0.08 per tablet
Lithium carbonate 300 mg		$8.13 for 100 capsules	$0.09 per capsule
Lithium carbonate	Eskalith® 300 mg	$15.25 for 100 capsules	$0.16 per capsule
	Eskalith® 300 mg	$15.25 for 100 tablets	$0.16 per tablet
	Eskalith CR® 450 mg	$32.30 for 100 tablets	$0.33 per tablet
	Lithonate® 300 mg	$7.00 for 100 capsules	$0.07 per capsule
	Lithane® 300 mg	$12.54 for 100 tablets	$0.13 per tablet
	Lithotabs® 300 mg	$6.89 for 100 tablets	$0.07 per tablet
Lithium citrate 8 mEq lithium per 5 ml (equivalent to 300 mg lithium carbonate)		$17.00 for 500 ml	$0.17 per 5 ml

* AWP is the average wholesale price to the pharmacist that is listed in the *1994 Redbook* (Cardinale, 1994).

REFERENCES

Alessi, N, Naylor, MW, Ghaziuddin, M, Zubieta, JK. Update on lithium carbonate therapy in children and adolescents. *J Am Acad Child Adolesc Psychiatry*, 1994;33:291-304.

Campbell, M, Gonzalez, NM, Silva, RR. The pharmacologic treatment of conduct disorders and rage outbursts. *Psych Clin North Amer,* 1992;15:69-85.

Campbell, M, Fish, B, Shapiro, T, Collins, P, Koh, C. Lithium and chlorpromazine: A controlled crossover study of hyperactive severely disturbed children. *J Autism Child Schizophrenia,* 1972;2:234-263.

Campbell, M, Small, AM, Green, WH, Jennings, SJ, Perry, R., Bennett, WG, Anderson, L. Behavioral efficacy of haloperidol and lithium carbonate: A comparison of hospitalized aggressive children with conduct disorder. *Arch Gen Psych,* 1984;41:650-656.

Campbell, M, Silva, RR, Kafantaris, V, Locascio, JJ, Gonzalez, NM, Lee, D, Lynch, NS. Predictors of side effects associated with lithium administration in children. *Psychopharm Bull,* 1991;27:373-380.

Cardinale, VA (ed). *1994 Drug Topics Redbook*, Medical Economics Company, Inc., 1994; 190, 254-255.

Cooper, TB, Bergner, PE, Simpson, GM. The 24-hour serum lithium level as a prognosticator of dosage requirement. *Am J Psych,* 1973;130:601-603.

Dale, PG. Lithium therapy in aggressive mentally subnormal patients. *Brit J Psych,* 1980;137:469-474.

DeLong, GR, Nieman, GW. Lithium-induced behavior changes in children with symptoms suggesting manic-depressive illness. *Psychopharm Bull,* 1983; 19:258-265.

DeLong, GR, Aldershof, AL. Long-term experience with lithium treatment in childhood: Correlation with clinical diagnosis. *J Amer Acad Child Adolesc Psychiatry,* 1987;26:389-394.

Dietrich, A, Mortensen, ME, Wheller, J. Cardiac toxicity in an adolescent following chronic lithium and imipramine therapy. *J Adolesc Health,* 1992;14: 394-397.

Dostal, T, Zvolsky, P. Anti-aggressive effect of lithium salts in severe mentally retarded adolescents. *International Pharmacopsychiatry,* 1970;5:203-207.

Fetner, HH, Geller, B. Lithium and tricyclic antidepressants. *Psych Clin North Amer,* 1992;15:223-241.

Geller, B, Fetner, HH. Children's 24-hour serum lithium level after a single dose predicts initial dose and steady-state plasma levels. *J Clin Psychopharm,* 1989; 9:155.

Himmelhoch, JM. On the failure to recognize lithium failure. *Psych Annals,* 1994;24:241-250.

Jefferson, JW, Greist, JH, Ackerman, DL, Caroll, JA. *Lithium Encyclopedia for Clinical Practice.* Washington: American Psychiatric Press, 1987.

Khandelwal, SK, Varma, VK, Murphy, RS. Renal function in children receiving long-term lithium prophylaxis. *Am J Psych,* 1984;141:278-279.

Physician's Desk Reference. Oradell, NJ: Medical Economic Data. 1994.

Platt, JE, Campbell, M, Green, WH, Grega, DM. Cognitive effects of lithium carbonate and haloperidol in treatment-resistant aggressive children. *Arch Gen Psych,* 1984;41:657-662.

Ryan, ND, Meyer, V, Dachille, S, Mazzie, D, Puig-Antich, J. Lithium antidepressant augmentation in TCA-refractory depression in adolescents. *J Amer Acad Child Adolesc Psychiatry,* 1988;27:371-376.

Shader, RI, Greenblatt, DJ. Practice guidelines and lithium levels. *J Clin Psychopharm,* 1992;12:303.

Silva, RR, Campbell, M, Golden, RR, Small, AM, Pataki, CS, Rosenberg, CR. Side effects associated with lithium and placebo administration in aggressive children. *Psychopharm Bull,* 1992;28:319-326.

Strober, M, Morrell, W, Lampert, C, Burroughs, J. Relapse following discontinuation of lithium maintenance therapy in adolescents with bipolar I illness: A naturalistic study. *Am J Psych,* 1990;147:457-461.

Strober, M, Freeman, R, Rigali, J, Schmidt, S, Diamond, R. The pharmacotherapy of depressive illness in adolescence: II. Effects of lithium augmentation in nonresponders to imipramine. *J Amer Acad Child Adolesc Psychiatry,* 1992; 31:16-20.

United States Pharmacopeia, Drug Information, 1994, Volumes I and II. Sections on lithium.

Varanka, TM, Weller, RA, Weller, EB, Fristad, MA. Lithium treatment of manic episodes with psychotic features in prepubertal children. *Am J Psych,* 1988; 145:1557-1559.

Vitiello, B, Behar, D, Malone, R, Delaney, MA, Ryan, PJ, Simpson, GM. Pharmacokinetics of lithium carbonate in children. *J Clin Psychopharm,* 1988;8: 355-359.

Weller, EB, Weller, RA, Fristad, MA. Lithium dosage guide for prepubertal children: A preliminary report. *J Amer Acad Child Psychiatry,* 1986;25:92-95.

Chapter 5

Benzodiazepines

Alprazolam

    Xanax® is marketed by UpJohn.

    Alprazolam is also available in generic form.

Chlordiazepoxide

    Librium® is marketed by Roche Laboratories.

    Chlordiazepoxide is also available in generic form.

Clonazepam

    Klonopin® is marketed by Roche Laboratories.

Diazepam

    Valium® is marketed by Roche Laboratories.

    Diazepam is also available in generic form.

Lorazepam

    Ativan® is marketed by Wyeth-Ayerst.

    Lorazepam is also available in generic form.

DSM-IV INDICATIONS

Anxiety Disorders (???)

Tic Disorders (???)

FDA: Safety and efficacy have not been established in patients less than 18 years of age for alprazolam. Chlordiazepoxide is not recommended for children less than six years of age. Diazepam is not for use in children less than six months of age. Lorazepam is not indicated for patients less than 12 years of age. Clonazepam is used in children and infants for seizure disorders (*PDR*, 1994).

USP: Children, especially the very young, are more sensitive to the CNS effects of benzodiazepines (*USPDI*, 1994).

CONTRAINDICATIONS: Hypersensitivity to benzodiazepines, personal substance abuse or family history of substance abuse, pregnancy, symptoms of impulsivity or aggression, psychosis or depression.

PHARMACOLOGY: The benzodiazepines appear to increase the effects of gamma-aminobutyrate (GABA) and other inhibitory neurotransmitters by binding to specific benzodiazepine receptors. Benzodiazepine receptors appear to be part of a membrane complex involving chloride channels and GABA receptors. GABA is the principal neurotransmitter in the brain. Benzodiazepines also affect the neurotransmitters serotonin, norepinephrine, and dopamine (Coffey, 1990). Benzodiazepine-induced increases in GABA activity result in disinhibition, reduction in arousal, anxiolytic, sedative, hypnotic, anticonvulsant and muscle relaxant effects (Kutcher et al., 1992).

STUDIES OF BENZODIAZEPINE EFFICACY

Anxiety

There is very limited data on the safety and efficacy of the benzodiazepines in children and adolescents, but they are frequently used to treat anxiety in this population (Simeon, 1993). The lack of drug efficacy studies for younger patients may be due to the lack of recognition of symptoms of anxiety, the heterogeneity of patients, lack of reliable assessment methods, and different opinions on the nature of childhood anxiety and its management (Simeon, 1993). The current anxiety disorders in children and adolescents include simple phobia, social phobia, avoidant disorder, separation anxiety, overanxious disorder, panic disorder (with or without agoraphobia), and post traumatic stress disorder. Kutcher et al. (1992) indicate that much work is needed to determine the diagnostic reliability, diagnostic validity, natural course, outcome, comorbidity, and treatment of the anxiety disorders. In addition, anxiety disorders frequently present with depression, substance abuse, attention-deficit/hyperactivity disorder, and other disorders (Kutcher et al., 1992). It is difficult to determine drug efficacy and safety in a such a heterogeneous population.

Several studies involving the use of low-potency benzodiazepines (chlordiazepoxide and diazepam) in children and adolescents were reported in the 1960s (Kutcher et al., 1992). Each study included a heterogeneous group of patients that had various diagnoses of school phobia, anxiety, school refusing, depression, phobias, psychoneurosis, and schizophrenia. The open studies suggest that chlordiazepoxide may be effective in the treatment of school refusal (D'Amato, 1962; Kraft et al., 1965). In these early studies, chlordiazepoxide doses of 10 to 60 mg per day and diazepam doses of 5 to 20 mg per day were utilized. Side effects reported include behavioral disinhibition, drowsiness, dizziness, and worsening of behavior. The diagnostic heterogeneity of the patients and the lack of proper research design make the early studies difficult to evaluate (Kutcher et al., 1992).

Bernstein, Garfinkel, and Borchardt (1990) reported two different trials of alprazolam in the treatment of school refusal. The first trial was an open study that included 17 children and adolescents (aged 9.5 to 17 years) that compared the effects of imipramine to alprazolam. Thirteen of the patients had symptoms of anxiety and depression, and four patients had symptoms of depression only. The mean dose of alprazolam used was 1.43 mg per day with a range of 0.75 to 4.0 mg per day. The mean dose of imipramine was 135 mg per day with a range of 50 to 175 mg per day. Six out of nine patients taking the alprazolam were rated as moderately to markedly improved in anxiety and depression. Four out of six patients taking imipramine were rated as moderately to markedly improved. A follow-up double-blind, placebo-controlled, eight-week study compared the effects of alprazolam, imipramine, and placebo. Twenty-four patients (aged 7.6 to 17.5 years, mean of 14.1 years) with school refusal were studied. Patients were diagnosed with depressive disorder (N = 10), anxiety disorder (N = 4), or a combination of depression and anxiety disorder (N = 10), and randomly assigned to alprazolam, imipramine, or placebo. In addition, each child participated in a school reentry plan. Results indicate there was no significant difference between the drug groups and placebo. Doses of alprazolam were 0.02 to 0.03 mg/kg/day (1.0 to 3.0 mg/ day). Doses of imipramine were 2.64 to 3.3 mg/kg/day (150 to 300 mg per day). Adverse effects that occurred more commonly with active treatment include blurred vision, constipation, dizziness, dizziness with standing, dry mouth, and nausea (Bernstein, Garfinkel, and Borchardt, 1990).

Simeon et al. (1992) reported a double-blind, placebo-controlled, four-week study of alprazolam in the treatment of children and adolescents with overanxious and avoidant disorder. The study included 30 patients (ages 8.4 to 16.9 years, mean age of 12.6 years). Alprazolam was administered in daily doses of 0.5 to 3.5 mg per day with a mean dose of 1.57 mg/day. The differences in therapeutic effect between alprazolam and placebo did not reach statistical significance. The medication was tolerated and the side effects of tiredness and dry mouth were reported equally for both the alprazolam and placebo. Rebound or withdrawal symptoms were not observed (Simeon et al., 1992).

Biederman (1987) reported three cases of anxiety disorders with panic-like symptoms that responded to clonazepam therapy. The patients were two eight-year-old boys and an 11-year-old girl. Clonazepam doses of 0.5 to 3.0 mg per day were utilized to treat the various symptoms of anxiety, and all patients improved with no clinically significant side effects. Kutcher and Mackenzie (1988) reported an open trial of four adolescents (aged 16 to 19) treated for panic attacks and anxiety symptoms with clonazepam 0.5 mg two times daily. The average frequency of the panic attacks was reduced from three per week to 0.25 per week. Drowsiness was the only reported side effect in this study. The preliminary results from a double-blind, placebo-controlled study of 12 adolescents with panic disorder suggest that clonazepam is more effective than placebo in reducing the number of panic attacks per week (Kutcher et al., 1992). Drowsiness was the most commonly reported side effect, but one patient on clonazepam dropped out due to increasing irritability and restlessness. A case report, by Ross and Piggott (1993) indicated that clonazepam 1.0 mg two times daily was helpful in the treatment-resistant case of a 14-year-old boy diagnosed with obsessive compulsive disorder.

Tic Disorders

Steingard et al. (1994) reported the clinical treatment of seven children and adolescents (aged seven to 13 years) with a tic disorder and concomitant attention-deficit/hyperactivity disorder (ADHD). Five of the patients also met the criteria for oppositional defiant or conduct disorder. Clonidine therapy resulted in a decrease in the symptoms of ADHD and the frequency of tics. The addition of clonazepam 0.25 to 2.0 mg per day resulted in a further decrease in tic frequency and severity without affecting the coexisting ADHD. Side effects included mild sedation that required the discontinuation of clonazepam in one patient.

DEVELOPMENTAL PHARMACOKINETICS

(Pharmacokinetic data are not available in children and adolescents.)

Absorption: Benzodiazepines are well absorbed from the gastrointestinal tract.
Onset of action: Therapeutic effects may occur within one week or sooner.
Metabolism: Children may have an increased ability to metabolize these drugs, requiring more frequent dosing.
Duration of action: Unknown.
Half-life: Unknown. Chlordiazepoxide, diazepam, and clonazepam have long half-lives (> 24 hours) in adults. Lorazepam and alprazolam have shorter half-lives (ten to 12 hours) in adults.
Plasma levels: Therapeutic blood levels have not been established in children, adolescents, or adults (Coffey, 1983; Coffey, 1990).

DOSAGE RANGES

Practitioners recommend that the initial dose of a benzodiazepine be small and dosage increments be made gradually. Titrations of the dose should be according to individual response and ability to tolerate adverse effects (Coffey, 1990; Kutcher et al., 1992). Children tend to have more efficient hepatic metabolism and renal excretion and require more frequent administration than adults. Benzodiazepines are administered in two to four divided daily doses to children. The duration of therapy should be individualized, however, Kutcher et al. (1992) recommend that in the treatment of anxiety, the medication may be continued for four to six months after which a drug-free trial is indicated.

> **Alprazolam:** Alprazolam is not approved for use in patients less than 18 years of age. In the studies described above alprazolam doses of 0.5 to 4.0 mg administered in divided daily doses were utilized (Bernstein, Garfinkel, and Borchardt, 1990; Simeon et al., 1992).
>
> **Chlordiazepoxide:** For children six years old and older, the initial dose is 5 mg and may be increased to a maximum of 30 mg per day administered in three divided doses.
>
> **Clonazepam:** Clonazepam is indicated in the treatment of seizures in children. In the studies described above, clonazepam doses of 0.5 to 3.0 mg per day were administered (Biederman, 1987; Kutcher and Mackenzie, 1988; Steingard et al., 1994).
>
> **Diazepam:** Diazepam doses range from 1.0 to 20 mg per day (Kutcher et al., 1992).
>
> **Lorazepam:** Lorazepam doses range from 0.25 to 4.0 mg per day (Kutcher et al., 1992).

ADVERSE EFFECTS REPORTED IN CHILDREN/ADOLESCENTS

COMMON

> Drowsiness and fatigue may require dosage adjustment. Other reported side effects are blurred vision, constipa-

tion, dizziness, dizziness with standing, dry mouth and nausea, irritability, restlessness, and worsening of behavior (Bernstein, Garfinkel, and Borchardt, 1990; Kutcher et al., 1992).

Cognitive/memory impairment: Although this particular side effect has not been evaluated in children or adolescents, the effect may be particularly troublesome for this population. In adults, benzodiazepines are associated with anterograde amnesia (short-term memory loss after drug administration). This particular side effect may affect the academic performance of a child or adolescent.

Behavioral disinhibition: Behavioral disinhibition can be a therapeutic effect and an adverse effect. This effect has been reported in children and adolescents (Reiter and Kutcher, 1991). For patients who are very inhibited this effect may allow more normal social activity. For the child or adolescent who is impulsive and not very inhibited the effect can be very disturbing. The adverse effect of behavioral disinhibition is manifested by excitation, agitation, aggression, hyperactivity, rage outbursts, and incoordination. The frequency of benzodiazepine-induced disinhibition as an adverse effect ranges from 0 to 30 percent (Coffey, 1990). Patients who are more likely to develop this adverse effect are younger, more impulsive, and mentally retarded (Coffey, 1990; Simeon, 1993). Treatment of behavioral disinhibition requires discontinuation of the medication and observation.

LESS COMMON

Due to the lack of extended treatment studies, there is a lack of information in this area. Practitioners are encouraged to monitor for the adverse effects that have been reported for adults, until further information is available.

Withdrawal: Abrupt discontinuation of benzodiazepine therapy is not recommended. Although benzodiazepine withdrawal has not been reported in children or adolescents, this is most likely due to the lack of reports of the use of benzodiazepines. Signs and symptoms reported in adults of abrupt benzodiazepine withdrawal include return of original symptoms, nausea, vomiting, anorexia, fatigue, restlessness, sweating, irritability, muscle tension/cramps, tremor, dysphoria, confusion, delusions, hallucinations, and seizures. Benzodiazepine therapy should be tapered over several days to weeks to avoid withdrawal effects.

Teratogenic effect: Benzodiazepines are associated with an increased risk of physical malformations and are contraindicated during pregnancy.

ALLERGIC REACTION: Skin rash or itching may occur requiring discontinuation of the medication. Hypersensitivity to one benzodiazepine indicates possible hypersensitivity to other benzodiazepines.

TOXICITY: Benzodiazepine toxicity is manifested by sleepiness, confusion, slurred speech, ataxia, trembling, decreased reflexes, slow pulse, shortness of breath, and coma. Respiratory depression, associated with benzodiazepine overdoses, is found more frequently in patients on polydrug therapy or who have concurrent illnesses.

DRUG INTERACTIONS

DRUG	DRUGS	EFFECT
Benzodiazepines	Alcohol, other medications that produce CNS depression	Enhanced central nervous system depression may occur. The use of alcohol should be discouraged.
Benzodiazepines	Antacids	Concurrent use will delay absorption, but not reduce the total amount of absorption.
Benzodiazepines	Tricyclic antidepressants	In addition to added CNS depression, alprazolam therapy is associated with increased blood levels of tricyclic antidepressants.

Benzodiazepines	Carbamazepine	Carbamazepine induces hepatic microsomal enzyme activity that may reduce the blood levels of the benzodiazepines.
Benzodiazepines	Cimetidine, Oral contraceptives, Erythromycin, Fluoxetine, Propranolol, Valproic acid	Concurrent use may increase blood levels of the benzodiazepines due to inhibition of hepatic metabolism. Monitoring and possible benzodiazepine dose reduction is indicated.
Benzodiazepines	Clozapine	Concurrent administration has resulted in collapse, respiratory depression or arrest. Concurrent administration is not recommended.
Benzodiazepines	Digoxin	Digoxin levels may be increased. Monitor serum levels of digoxin.
Benzodiazepines	Phenytoin	Phenytoin levels may be increased. Monitor serum levels of phenytoin.
Benzodiazepines	Zidovudine	Due to competition for hepatic enzymes, the clearance of zidovudine may be decreased resulting in increased zidovudine toxicity.

MONITORING GUIDELINES

Baseline Assessment:

- History and physical, including weight and height of the patient.
- Pregnancy test for females with child-bearing potential.
- Complete blood count, liver, and renal function tests.

Time Pattern for Response:

- Anti-anxiety effects may be observed within one week or sooner. Dosage adjustments may be necessary to receive full benefit.

Follow-Up Assessment

- Monitor for signs and symptoms of agranulocytosis or other blood dyscrasias including infections, fever, unusual tiredness, or weakness. Repeat complete blood count if indicated.
- Monitor for memory impairment or paradoxical reactions (hallucinations, insomnia, unusual excitement, irritability). Monitor for signs and symptoms of overdose including sedation, confusion, shakiness, shortness of breath, slurred speech, and ataxia.
- Assess therapeutic response and need for continued therapy.

Drug Discontinuation:

- Abrupt withdrawal of benzodiazepines is not recommended in any population of patients. Signs and symptoms of abrupt withdrawal include return of anxiety, insomnia, irritability, shakiness, tremors, sweating, body aches and pains, muscle cramps, vomiting, seizures, delirium, and psychosis. It is suggested by Coffey (1990) that children may be at higher risk of seizures associated with benzodiazepine withdrawal than adults. Children may have a faster metabolic clearance of the benzodiazepines and more neurodevelopmental abnormalities. The dose of benzodiazepines should be gradually tapered over several weeks and occasionally longer (Coffey, 1990; Kutcher et al., 1992). Dangers of withdrawal may be greater with the shorter-acting benzodiazepines–alprazolam and lorazepam. Withdrawal phenomenon have not been reported in children or adolescents (Coffey, 1990; Kutcher et al., 1992).

SPECIAL INSTRUCTIONS FOR PARENTS/CARE GIVERS/ CHILDREN/ADOLESCENTS

- Benzodiazepines may cause drowsiness during the first few weeks of therapy. If this happens, the patient should not participate in activities that require alertness, such as riding a bike or driving a car.

• Alcohol and other depressants are to be avoided during therapy with a benzodiazepine.

• Check with your physician or pharmacist before taking any other drugs. Be sure to tell all physicians, pharmacists, and dentists that you are taking a benzodiazepine.

• Do not abruptly stop taking this medication; withdrawal symptoms may occur. Benzodiazepine therapy needs to be decreased slowly under the direction of a physician.

• Sometimes patients have the opposite reaction to a benzodiazepine causing the patient's symptoms to become worse. If the patient develops excitement, irritability, anger, aggression, uncontrollable behavior, or memory loss, stop the medication and call the physician.

• Report to the physician any signs of side effects to the benzodiazepines including sore throat or other infections, persistent tiredness, sedation, yellow eyes or skin, and any other unusual reaction.

• Patients who are pregnant should not take benzodiazepines.

• Store this medication and all medications away from the patient and other children and adolescents.

PRODUCTS AVAILABLE

Alprazolam is marketed as Xanax® by UpJohn. Xanax® is available is 0.25, 0.5, 1.0, and 2.0 mg tablets. Xanax® 0.25 mg is a white, scored, oval tablet imprinted with Xanax 29. Xanax® 0.5 mg is a peach, scored, oval tablet imprinted with Xanax 55. Xanax® 1.0 mg is a lavender, scored, oval tablet imprinted with Xanax 90. Xanax® 2.0 mg is a white, multi-scored, oblong tablet imprinted with Xanax 90. Alprazolam is also available in generic form in the same dosage strengths.

Chlordiazepoxide is marketed as Librium® by Roche Laboratories. Librium® is available in 5, 10, and 25 mg capsules. Librium® 5 mg is a green and yellow capsule imprinted with Librium 5 Roche. Librium® 10 mg is a green and black capsule imprinted with Librium 10 Roche. Librium® 25 mg is a green and white capsule imprinted with Librium 25 Roche. Chlordiazepoxide is also available in generic form in the same dosage strengths.

Clonazepam is marketed as Klonopin® by Roche Laboratories. Klonopin® is available in 0.5, 1.0, and 2.0 mg tablets. Klonopin® 0.5 mg is an orange, scored tablet imprinted with Roche and Klonopin. Klonopin® 1.0 mg is a blue, scored tablet imprinted with Roche and Klonopin 1. Klonopin® 2.0 mg is a white, scored tablet imprinted with Roche and Klonopin 2.

Diazepam is marketed as Valium® by Roche Laboratories. Valium® is available in 2, 5, and 10 mg tablets. Valium® 2 mg is a white, scored tablet, with a cut-out V design, imprinted with Roche 2 Valium. Valium® 5 mg is a yellow, scored tablet, with a cut-out V design, imprinted with Roche 5 Valium. Valium® 10 mg is a blue, scored tablet, with a cut-out V design, imprinted with Roche 10 Valium. Diazepam is also available in generic form in the same dosage strengths.

Lorazepam is marketed as Ativan® by Wyeth-Ayerst. Ativan® is available in 0.5, 1.0, and 2.0 mg tablets. Ativan® 0.5 mg is a white, five-sided, scored tablet imprinted with a raised A/Wyeth 81. Ativan® 1.0 mg is a white, five-sided, scored tablet imprinted with a raised A/Wyeth 64. Ativan® 2.0 mg is a white, five-sided, scored tablet imprinted with a raised A/Wyeth 65. Lorazepam is also available in generic form in the same dosage strengths.

COST

GENERIC NAME	TRADENAME	AWP*	AWP* per dose
Alprazolam 0.25 mg		$48.20 for 100 tablets	$0.49 per tablet
Alprazolam 0.50 mg		$60.12 for 100 tablets	$0.61 per tablet
Alprazolam 1.0 mg		$80.22 for 100 tablets	$0.81 per tablet
Alprazolam 2.0 mg		$136.20 for 100 tablets	$1.37 per tablet
Alprazolam	Xanax® 0.25 mg	$59.98 for 100 tablets	$0.60 per tablet

	Xanax® 0.5 mg	$73.09 for 100 tablets	$0.74 per tablet
	Xanax® 1.0 mg	$94.86 for 100 tablets	$0.95 per tablet
	Xanax® 2.0 mg	$153.13 for 100 tablets	$1.54 per tablet
Chlordiazepoxide 5 mg		$5.05 for 100 capsules	$0.06 per capsule
Chlordiazepoxide 10 mg		$5.20 for 100 capsules	$0.06 per capsule
Chlordiazepoxide 25 mg		$5.40 for 100 capsules	$0.06 per capsule
Chlordiazepoxide	Librium® 5 mg	$35.53 for 100 capsules	$0.36 per capsule
	Librium® 10 mg	$50.60 for 100 capsules	$0.51 per capsule
	Librium® 25 mg	$84.99 for 100 capsules	$0.85 per capsule
Clonazepam	Klonopin® 0.5 mg	$67.28 for 100 tablets	$0.68 per tablet
	Klonopin® 1.0 mg	$76.36 for 100 tablets	$0.77 per tablet
	Klonopin® 2.0 mg	$104.62 for 100 tablets	$1.05 per tablet
Diazepam 2 mg		$4.95 for 100 tablets	$0.05 per tablet
Diazepam 5 mg		$6.85 for 100 tablets	$0.07 per tablet
Diazepam 10 mg		$11.50 for 100 tablets	$0.12 per tablet
	Valium® 2 mg	$36.48 for 100 tablets	$0.37 per tablet
	Valium® 5 mg	$56.74 for 100 tablets	$0.57 per tablet
	Valium® 10 mg	$95.61 for 100 tablets	$0.96 per tablet
Lorazepam 0.5 mg		$13.10 for 100 tablets	$0.14 per tablet
Lorazepam 1.0 mg		$16.30 for 100 tablets	$0.17 per tablet
Lorazepam 2.0 mg		$23.70 for 100 tablets	$0.24 per tablet
Lorazepam	Ativan® 0.5 mg	$53.89 for 100 tablets	$0.54 per tablet
	Ativan® 1.0 mg	$70.16 for 100 tablets	$0.71 per tablet
	Ativan® 2.0 mg	$102.30 for 100 tablets	$1.03 per tablet

* AWP is the average wholesale price to the pharmacist that is listed in the *1994 Redbook* (Cardinale, 1994).

REFERENCES

Bernstein, GA, Garfinkel, BD, Borchardt, CM. Comparative studies of pharmacotherapy for school refusal. *J Amer Acad Child Adolesc Psychiatry*, 1990; 29:773-781.

Biederman, J. Clonazepam in the treatment of prepubertal children with panic-like symptoms. *J Clin Psych,* 1987;48:38-41.

Cardinale, VA (ed). *1994 Drug Topics Redbook*, Medical Economic Company, Inc., 1994; 92, 109 136, 167, 246, 251, 256, 404, 413.

Coffey, BJ. Anxiolytics for children and adolescents: Traditional and new drugs. *J Child Adolesc Psychopharmacology,* 1990;1:57-83.

Coffey, B, Shader, RI, Greenblatt, DJ. Pharmacokinetics of benzodiazepines and psychostimulants in children. *J Clin Psychopharm,* 1983;3:217-225.

D'Amato, G. Chlordiazepoxide in management of school phobia. *Dis Nerv System*, 1962;139:1059-1060.

Kraft, IA. A clinical study of chlordiazepoxide used in psychiatric disorders of children. *International J Neuropsychiatry*, 1965;1: 433-437.

Kutcher, S, Mackenzie, S. Successful clonazepam treatment of adolescents with panic disorder. *J Clin Psychopharmacology*, 1988;8:299-301.

Kutcher, SP, Reiter, S, Gardner, DM, Klein, RG. The pharmacotherapy of anxiety disorders in children and adolescents. *Psych Clinic North Amer*, 1992;15: 41-67.

Physician's Desk Reference. Oradell, NJ: Medical Economic Data. 1994.

Reiter, S, Kutcher, SP. Disinhibition and anger outbursts in adolescents treated with clonazepam. *J Clin Psychopharmacology*, 1991;11:268.

Ross, DC, Piggott, LR. Clonazepam for OCD. *J Amer Acad Child Adolesc Psychiatry*, 1993;32:470-471.

Simeon, JG. Use of anxiolytics in children. *Encephale*, 1993;19:71-74.

Simeon, JG, Ferguson, HB, Knott, V. Clinical, cognitive and neurophysiologic effects of alprazolam in children and adolescents with overanxious and avoidant disorders. *J Amer Acad Child Adolesc Psychiatry*, 1992;31:29-33.

Steingard, RJ, Goldberg, M, Lee, D, DeMaso, DR. Adjunctive clonazepam treatment of tic symptoms in children with comorbid tic disorders and ADHD. *J Amer Acad Child Adolesc Psychiatry*, 1994;33:394-399.

United States Pharmacopeia, Drug Information, 1994, Volumes I and II. Sections on benzodiazepines.

Chapter 6

Other Agents Used in Child and Adolescent Psychiatry

BETA-BLOCKERS

Metoprolol

> Lopressor® is marketed by Geigy Pharmaceuticals.
>
> Metoprolol is also available in generic form.

Propranolol hydrochloride

> Inderal® is marketed by Wyeth-Ayerst.
>
> Propranolol is also available in generic form.

DSM-IV INDICATIONS

Anxiety (???)

Mental Retardation, aggression (???)

> FDA: For metoprolol, safety and efficacy in children have not been established. For propranolol, safety and efficacy have not been evaluated, but the information is available from the medical literature to allow fair estimates and specific dosing information for the treatment of cardiac diseases (*PDR*, 1994).
>
> USP: The use of beta-blocking agents in the pediatric population has not demonstrated pediatric-specific problems that limit the usefulness of these medications in children (*USPDI*, 1994).

CONTRAINDICATIONS: Hypersensitivity to propranolol or metoprolol; bronchospastic disease, asthma; bradycardia, cardiac arrhythmias, cardiovascular disease; diabetes or other disorders with hypoglycemia; hyperthyroidism; pheochromocytoma; electrolyte abnormalities, hepatic or renal function impairment; muscle weakness; allergen immunotherapy or allergenic extracts for skin testing; psoriasis; pregnancy; concurrent drug therapy (*see* Drug Interactions).

PHARMACOLOGY: Beta-blockers act as antagonists of norepinephrine and epinephrine at beta adrenergic receptors and have been used for a variety of cardiovascular disorders. The beta adrenergic receptors are divided into two types, beta-1 and beta-2. In general, beta-1 receptors are located in the heart and brain, and beta-2 receptors are located in the vascular, bronchial, and gastrointestinal systems. Propranolol and metoprolol are highly lipophilic beta-blockers that have both central and peripheral activity. Propranolol is nonselective and blocks both beta-1 and beta-2 receptors. Metoprolol is selective for beta-1 receptors, however, selectivity for a receptor is not absolute and metoprolol may block beta-2 receptors, especially at higher doses. Propranolol also antagonizes central serotonin receptors. The mechanism of action of the beta-blockers in treating anxiety or aggression is not known (Arnold and Aman, 1991).

The cardiovascular effects of propranolol and metoprolol are hypotension and bradycardia. Beta-blockers may also cause bronchospasm in patients with asthma, increase hypoglycemia, and cause a variety of central nervous system effects including psychosis, insomnia, hallucinations, fatigue and depression (Arnold and Aman, 1991). Propranolol inhibits the activity of the cytochrome P450 enzyme system that results in several drug interactions. The inhibition of this metabolic system by propranolol results in increased blood levels of neuroleptics, antidepressants, and numerous other medications.

STUDIES OF PROPRANOLOL EFFICACY

Anxiety

Famularo, Kinscherff, and Fenton (1988) reported a four-week open trial of propranolol therapy in 11 children aged six to 12 years.

Each of the children were in the acute stages of post traumatic stress disorder (PTSD). Acute PTSD is defined as having an onset of symptoms within six months of the trauma and a duration of symptoms less than six months. Children with mental retardation, schizophrenia, major depression, asthma, bradycardia, hypotension, hyperthyroidism, or pervasive developmental disorder were not included in the study. Propranolol was initiated at 0.8 mg/kg/day and was administered in three divided doses. Doses were increased to a maximum of 2.5 mg/kg/day. Dosage was titrated to a diastolic blood pressure of 55 mm Hg or a pulse rate of 55 beats per minute. The authors report significant improvement in affective, cognitive, and physiological symptoms of PTSD. Each patient improved while taking propranolol and became worse when treatment was discontinued. For three patients, doses of propranolol were limited by sedation, mild hypotension and lowered heart rate. The authors acknowledge that some of the positive effects of propranolol may be due to a placebo effect (Famularo, Kinscherff, and Fenton, 1988).

Van Winter and Stickler (1984) reported the case of a 12-year-old boy who began to have panic attacks at the age of eight years. Physical, laboratory, and electroencephalogram findings were within normal limits. Imipramine failed to treat the panic attacks, and propranolol 120 mg/day was administered. The patient initially responded to the propranolol, but the panic attacks returned within two months. The dose was increased to 160 mg per day and the patient continues to have a partial response. Garland and Smith (1990) reported a case of a 15-year-old boy in which propranolol therapy (dose was not specified) was unsuccessful in treating panic attacks. Based on these preliminary case reports, the effectiveness of propranolol for children with panic attacks appears to be minimal or absent.

Kymissis and Martin (1990) reported the successful use of propranolol to treat stuttering in a 15-year-old boy. The patient had a five year history of stuttering and responded to propranolol 10 mg daily. The effects of propranolol in this case could be attributed to an anti-anxiety, anti-stuttering, or a placebo response. These preliminary case reports require replication with more participants in order to determine the effects of propranolol in the treatment of anxiety disorders in children and adolescents.

Aggression

Williams et al. (1982) reported a 75 percent response rate in 30 patients (11 children, 15 adolescents, and four adults) who were treated with a one month trial of propranolol for treatment resistant uncontrolled rage outbursts. This open trial included a diagnostically heterogeneous group of patients with organic brain dysfunction. Patients with pervasive developmental disorder, conduct disorder with aggression, intermittent explosive disorder, severe uncontrolled seizures, and attention-deficit disorder with and without hyperactivity were included. During the trial, patients continued on their current medication regimens including antipsychotics, anticonvulsants, stimulants, or combinations of these agents. Propranolol was initiated at 30 to 80 mg per day in three to four divided doses. Doses were increased by 30 to 80 mg every three to seven days and dose titration was guided by side effects. The optimal dosing range is reported as 50 to 960 mg per day with a median dose of 161 mg per day. Reported side effects include sedation, hypotension, bradycardia (this patient took a double dose of propranolol or 320 mg), depression, wheezing, and dyspnea. The authors note that a wide range of optimal doses were observed in this study. This study is very difficult to interpret due to the use of multiple drugs. Propranolol interferes with the metabolism of several psychotropic and anticonvulsant medications resulting in increased blood levels of these drugs. Without adjustments in the doses or monitoring of the plasma levels of the psychotropics or anticonvulsants, it is very possible that propranolol increased the blood levels and activity of these medications.

Kuperman and Stewart (1987) reported an open trial of 16 patients, ages four to 24 years, treated with propranolol for physically aggressive behavior. The trial included a diagnostically heterogeneous group of patients with autism, mental retardation, attention-deficit disorder, and undersocialized aggressive conduct disorder. Patients at the beginning of the propranolol trial were taking other medications including neuroleptics, stimulants, or phenytoin. With the exception of the patient taking phenytoin, the other medications were discontinued over the three month trial of propranolol. Propranolol was initiated at doses of 20 mg two times daily and increased every four days according to response and cardiovascular effects. Doses were limited by a standing systolic blood pressure of 90 mm Hg, a diastolic blood pressure of 60 mm Hg, or a resting pulse of 60 beats per minute. Doses of propranolol ranged from 80 to 280 mg per day with a mean of 164 mg per day. Ten out of the 16 patients were rated by the teachers, parents, and physicians to be moderately or much improved, including six of the eight patients with mental retardation. The authors suggest that patients with mental retardation may have an increased response to propranolol and that nonresponders as a group appeared to be more sensitive to bradycardia associated with propranolol, thus limiting the dose administered (Kuperman and Stewart, 1987).

Grizenko and Vida (1988) reported the cases of two 12-year-old boys who responded to propranolol 50 mg three times daily. Each patient was highly aggressive but did not show signs of organic brain dysfunction. Propranolol was effective in reducing the rage reactions in both patients. Reported side effects were mild fatigue and hypotension. Matthews-Ferrai and Karroum (1992) reported an 11-year-old boy with asthma who was successfully treated with metoprolol for aggression. Metoprolol 25 mg three times daily reduced the frequency of outbursts. No side effects were reported. Kastner, Burlingham, and Friedman (1990) reported a 16-year-old boy with severe mental retardation, autism, and cerebral palsy who was noted to display perseveration, impulsivity, anxiety, and aggressive behavior when frustrated. The aggressive episodes occurred several times a day, were directed at care givers, and occasionally did not appear to have a precipitating factor. Metoprolol 40 mg per day was added to alprazolam 0.5 mg per day. The dose of metoprolol was increased to a maximum of 200 mg per day. The addition of metoprolol reduced the aggressive and impulsive behaviors. It is difficult to determine the effects of the metoprolol with concurrent administration of alprazolam. In this case report, it is possible that metoprolol treated alprazolam-induced behavioral disinhibition and may not have been effective alone.

DEVELOPMENTAL PHARMACOKINETICS

(Pharmacokinetic studies have not been conducted in children or adolescents.)

Absorption: Metoprolol and propranolol are completely absorbed with oral bioavailabilities of 30 to 50 percent.
Duration of action: Unknown. Doses are usually administered two to four times per day.
Half-life: In adults, the half-life of propranolol is three to five hours and the half-life of metoprolol is three to seven hours.
Plasma levels: Plasma levels have not been fully evaluated and are not clinically useful.

DOSAGE RANGES

Dosage adjustments are based on response and are limited by adverse effects including bradycardia and hypotension. Treatment studies have used the limits of standing systolic blood pressure of 90 mm Hg, diastolic blood pressure of 60 mm Hg, or a pulse of 60 beats per minute (Kuperman and Stewart, 1987). If hypotension or bradycardia occur, the next dose of the beta-blocker should be skipped and the total daily dose reassessed and reduced. Arnold and Aman (1991) suggest that lower doses of beta-blockers be initiated in children with mental retardation or developmental disorders. These children may be more sensitive to the effects of the beta-blockers. For the treatment of cardiac diseases in children, the doses of propranolol range from 2 to 4 mg/kg/day administered in two divided doses with a maximum of 16 mg/kg/day (Inderal® product information, Wyeth-Ayerst).

> **Aggression:** The average dose of propranolol used to treat aggression is 160 mg per day (Williams et al., 1982; Kuperman and Stewart, 1987), with a range of 80 to 280 mg per day (Kuperman and Stewart, 1987). Divided doses were administered three or four times daily. In two reported case studies, doses of metoprolol ranged from 75 to 200 mg per day administered in divided doses

(Matthews-Ferrai and Karroum, 1992; Kastner, Burlingham, and Friedman, 1990).

Anxiety: Famularo, Kinsherff, and Fenton (1988) used propranolol doses up to 2.5 mg/kg/day to treat post traumatic stress disorder.

ADVERSE EFFECTS REPORTED IN CHILDREN AND ADOLESCENTS

COMMON

The adverse effects reported in the preliminary studies described above include sedation, fatigue, bradycardia, hypotension, depression, wheezing, and dyspnea.

Cardiovascular effects: Doses of a beta-blocker are limited by bradycardia and hypotension. Guidelines used in the above studies recommend holding the dose of a beta-blocker if the pulse is less than 60 beats per minute, systolic blood pressure is less than 90 mm Hg, or diastolic blood pressure is less than 60 mm Hg. Subsequent doses of the beta-blocker should be reduced.

Respiratory: If symptoms of asthma, wheezing, or dyspnea occur, stop the medication. A specific beta-1 agent may or may not cause less respiratory symptoms.

Hypoglycemia: If hypoglycemia develops, discontinue the beta-blocker.

Depression or dysthymia: If symptoms of irritability, fatigue, or lethargy occur, reduce the dose or discontinue therapy.

LESS COMMON

Due to the lack of extended treatment studies, there is a lack of information in this area. Practitioners are encouraged to monitor for the numerous adverse effects that have been reported for adults until further information is available. Beta-blockers are associated with cardiovascular, psychiatric, endocrine, genitourinary, hematological, derma-tologic, ophthalmic, respiratory, musculoskeletal, etc., adverse effects.

ALLERGIC REACTION: Signs and symptoms of an allergic reaction in adults include: pharyngitis, photosensitivity reaction, erythematous rash, fever combined with aching and sore throat, laryngospasm, respiratory distress, or angioedema. Signs of an anaphylactic reaction include profound hypotension, bradycardia with or without atrioventricular nodal block, severe bronchospasm, hives, and angioedema.

TOXICITY: The manifestations of beta-blocker toxicity include: bradycardia, hypotension, cardiac arrhythmias, hypoglycemia, hyperkalemia, depressed consciousness, respiratory depression, bronchospasm, seizures, and coma.

DRUG INTERACTIONS

(Please note: There are numerous reported drug interactions with beta-blockers and only those drugs commonly used in children and adolescents are included here.)

DRUG	DRUGS	EFFECT
Beta-blockers	Aluminum salts, Calcium salts, Barbiturates, Nonsteroidal anti-inflammatory agents, Penicillins, Salicylates	Concurrent use may decrease the bioavailability and plasma levels of beta-blockers.
Beta-blockers	Oral contraceptives	Increased bioavailability and effects of the beta-blockers may occur.
Beta-blockers	Haloperidol, Phenothiazines	Pharmacological effects of both drugs may be increased.
Beta-blockers	Benzodiazepines	Increased effects of the benzodiazepines may occur.

Beta-blockers	Tricyclic antidepressants	Propranolol may inhibit the metabolism and increase blood levels (Gillette and Tannery, 1994).
Beta-blockers	Clonidine	Life-threatening and fatal increases in blood pressure have occurred after discontinuation of clonidine in patients receiving a beta-blocker or after simultaneous withdrawal.
Beta-blockers	Theophylline	Reduced elimination of theophylline may occur; monitoring of theophylline levels is indicated.
Beta-blockers	Cimetidine, Quinolones	Increased beta-blocker effect due to cimetidine induced inhibition of metabolism.
Beta-blockers	Monoamine oxidase inhibitors	Bradycardia may develop; concurrent use is not recommended.
Beta-blockers	Acetaminophen	Increased levels of acetaminophen may occur due to decreased clearance.
Beta-blockers	Anticoagulants	Propranolol may increase the anticoagulant effect of warfarin.
Beta-blockers	Antidiabetic agents or insulin	Beta-blockers may cause hyperglycemia and mask the symptoms of hypoglycemia. Concurrent use is not recommended.
Beta-blockers	Tobacco smoking	Tobacco smoking increases the metabolism of the beta-blockers and decreases the serum concentrations of beta-blockers. Cessation of tobacco smoking may result in the opposite effect with increased serum concentrations and effect of the beta-blockers.

Beta-blockers   Sympathomimetics   Concurrent use may inhibit the positive cardiovascular effects of the beta-blockers. The effects of this interaction in the treatment of anxiety or aggression is unknown.

MONITORING GUIDELINES

Baseline Assessment:

- History and physical, including weight and height of the patient.
- Blood pressure and pulse, electrocardiogram, electrolytes (serum sodium, glucose), and liver function tests. Other laboratory tests as indicated.
- Rule out contraindications to beta-blocker therapy (*see* Contraindications).

Time Pattern for Response:

- Therapeutic effect occurs within one to eight weeks.

Follow-Up Assessment:

- Limitations on dosage increases include a standing systolic blood pressure of 90 mm Hg, a diastolic blood pressure of 60 mm Hg, or a pulse of 60 beats per minute (Sylvester, 1993). Blood pressure and pulse should be monitored according to dose increases. Follow-up electrocardiograms have not been conducted in the preliminary investigations, but should be conducted in susceptible patients or in patients presenting with cardiovascular effects.
- Monitor for the possibility of adverse effects reported in adult patients including cardiovascular, psychiatric, endocrine, genitourinary, hematological, dermatologic, ophthalmic, respiratory, musculoskeletal, etc., adverse effects.
- Monitor for drug interactions (*see* Drug Interactions).
- After the patient has been successfully maintained for a substantial period of time, consider tapering the dose and reassessing response. If the patient tolerates the reduction consider further reductions and slowly discontinue the drug (Arnold and Aman, 1991).

Drug Discontinuation:

- Abrupt withdrawal of beta-blockers is not recommended. Gradual decreases in the dose over one to two weeks is recommended (Inderal®, product information, Wyeth-Ayerst). For adult patients, gradual tapering of the dose is done to avoid rebound hypertension, angina, and ventricular arrhythmias. While it is less likely that healthy children or adolescents will have an adverse cardiovascular effect, gradual tapering is recommended for all patients.

SPECIAL INSTRUCTIONS FOR PARENTS/CARE GIVERS/CHILDREN/ADOLESCENTS

- Be sure to tell the physician if you have asthma, diabetes, thyroid problems, or heart problems.
- Beta-blockers may cause drowsiness, dizziness, or blurred vision during the first few weeks of therapy. If this happens, the patient should not participate in activities that require alertness, such as riding a bike or driving a car.
- Be sure to call your physician if any of the following side effects occur: tiredness, slow pulse rate, dizziness, lightheadedness, confusion or depression, skin rash, fever, sore throat, unusual bleeding, or bruising.
- Beta-blockers can lower blood pressure and pulse. The physician will want to measure the blood pressure and pulse routinely while doses are adjusted.
- Do not stop using propranolol without contacting your physician. Your physician will want to reduce the dose of propranolol slowly. Abruptly stopping propranolol may result in large increases in blood pressure and other unwanted effects.
- Be sure to tell all physicians, pharmacists, and dentists that this medication is being taken. Do not take any other medication without checking with your physician or pharmacist.
- Taking metoprolol or propranolol with food will increase the amount of drug in the blood. Be sure to take the medication with food at the same time every day.

• Store this medication and all medications away from the patient and other children and adolescents.

PRODUCTS AVAILABLE

Metoprolol is available as Lopressor® from Geigy Pharmaceuticals and is available as a generic product. Propranolol hydrochloride is available as Inderal® from Wyeth-Ayerst and is available as a generic product.

Lopressor® is marketed in 50 mg pink, scored, capsule-shaped, tablets imprinted with Geigy 51 51. Lopressor® 100 mg is a light blue, scored, capsule-shaped, biconvex tablet imprinted with Geigy 71 71. Metoprolol is also available in the same dosage strengths as a generic product.

Inderal® is marketed in 10 mg peach, hexagonal, scored tablets imprinted with Inderal 10. Inderal® 20 mg is a blue, hexagonal, scored tablet imprinted with Inderal 20. Inderal® 40 mg is a green, hexagonal, scored tablet imprinted with Inderal 40. Inderal® 60 mg is a pink, hexagonal, scored tablet imprinted with Inderal 60. Inderal® 80 mg is a yellow, hexagonal, scored tablet imprinted with Inderal 80. Propranolol hydrochloride is also available in the same dosage strengths as a generic product.

COST

GENERIC NAME	TRADENAME	AWP*	AWP* per dose
Propranolol 10 mg		$1.20 for 100 tablets	$0.02 per tablet
Propranolol 20 mg		$1.65 for 100 tablets	$0.02 per tablet
Propranolol 40 mg		$3.24 for 100 tablets	$0.04 per tablet
Propranolol 60 mg		$2.25 for 100 tablets	$0.03 per tablet
Propranolol 80 mg		$2.55 for 100 tablets	$0.03 per tablet
Propranolol	Inderal® 10 mg	$27.89 for 100 tablets	$0.28 per tablet
	Inderal® 20 mg	$39.15 for 100 tablets	$0.40 per tablet
	Inderal® 40 mg	$41.43 for 100 tablets	$0.42 per tablet
	Inderal® 60 mg	$70.28 for 100 tablets	$0.71 per tablet
	Inderal® 80 mg	$77.99 for 100 tablets	$0.78 per tablet

Metoprolol 50 mg		$43.50 for 100 tablets	$0.44 per tablet
Metoprolol 100 mg		$65.40 for 100 tablets	$0.66 per tablet
Metoprolol	Lopressor® 50 mg	$47.57 for 100 tablets	$0.48 per tablet
	Lopressor® 100 mg	$74.59 for 100 tablets	$0.75 per tablet

* AWP is the average wholesale price to the pharmacist that is listed in the *1994 Redbook* (Cardinale, 1994).

BUSPIRONE

Buspirone hydrochloride

Buspar® is marketed by Mead Johnson.

DSM-IV INDICATIONS

Aggression (???)

Anxiety (???)

Autism (???)

> FDA: Safety and efficacy have not been established in pediatric populations (*PDR,* 1994).
> USP: Appropriate studies on the relationship of age to the effects of buspirone have not been performed in children up to 18 years of age (*USPDI,* 1994).

CONTRAINDICATIONS: Hypersensitivity to buspirone, pregnancy, and hepatic or renal dysfunction.

PHARMACOLOGY: Buspirone, an azaspirodecanedione, is an anti-anxiety agent that is not chemically related to the benzodiazepines, barbiturates, neuroleptics, or tricyclic antidepressants. Buspirone does not interact with benzodiazepine/GABA receptor complex and does not have anticonvulsant or muscle relaxant effects. Buspirone has multiple effects in the central nervous system. Buspirone has serotonin (5HT1A) agonist activity and interacts as an agonist and an antagonist at dopamine-2 receptors. In contrast to other anxiolytics, buspirone increases the firing rate of norepinephrine in the locus ceruleus and is not associated with impairment of psychomotor or cognitive skills. There is no evidence that buspirone is associated with physical or psychological abuse or dependence. Buspirone produces a dose-dependent increase in prolactin secretion. The effects of buspirone have not been fully evaluated in children or adolescents.

STUDIES OF BUSPIRONE EFFICACY

Aggression

Quiason, Ward, and Kitchen (1991) reported a case report of an eight-year-old boy with conduct disorder and attention-deficit/hyperactivity disorder (ADHD). The patient had a history of unprovoked aggressive and assaultive behavior. Buspirone was initiated at 5 mg three times a day and was increased to 15 mg three times a day. The authors noted a gradual reduction and cessation of aggressive behavior over ten days of therapy. Buspirone did not modify the symptoms of ADHD. No side effects were reported.

Anxiety

Kranzler (1988) reported a case of a 13-year-old boy with school refusal who was diagnosed with overanxious disorder. The patient complained of considerable anxiety and had primary nocturnal enuresis. He was initially treated with desipramine up to 125 mg per day. Desipramine therapy resulted in constipation and an elevated pulse rate and was discontinued. Several months later the patient was started on buspirone 2.5 mg three times a day that was subsequently increased to 5 mg three times daily. On the higher dose the patient experienced drowsiness, and the dose was lowered to 5 mg two times daily. The patient tolerated the buspirone and appeared to be significantly less anxious. Buspirone was not effective in treating the enuresis.

A case report by Alessi and Bos (1991) described an 11-year-old girl with a four-year-history of obsessive-compulsive disorder and six-month history of depression. The patient was initially treated with imipramine that resulted in cardiovascular side effects. Imipramine was discontinued, and fluoxetine was initiated and increased to 60 mg per day. Augmentation with trazodone resulted in sedation and was replaced with buspirone 10 mg per day increased to 30 mg per day. This combination decreased her depression and there was improvement in obsessive-compulsiveness. No side effects were reported.

Simeon (1993) reported the preliminary results of an open trial of buspirone in 13 patients (aged six to 14 years). The study included a heterogeneous group of patients with diagnoses of separation anxiety, overanxious disorder with and without attention-deficit/hyperactivity disorder, avoidant disorder, and obsessive-compulsive disorder. The parents reported additional symptoms of panic attacks, depression, and migraine headaches. Placebo was administered for two weeks followed by four weeks of buspirone therapy. The maximum daily dose of buspirone is 20 mg per day. Improvement was marked in two patients and moderate in ten patients. Buspirone therapy resulted in decreased anxiety and depression. Adverse effects in this study were rated as mild and transient, and included sleep difficulties, tiredness, nausea, stomach pains, and headaches. This open study (Simeon, 1993) and the above case reports suggest that much more work needs to be done in this area.

Autism

Realmuto, August, and Garfinkel (1989) reported the effects of buspirone in comparison to fenfluramine or methylphenidate in four children (aged nine to ten years) with autistic disorder. In this open trial, buspirone was administered for four weeks at doses up to 5 mg three times daily. After four weeks of buspirone and a one-week washout, patients were switched to methylphenidate or fenfluramine up to 20 mg per day for either drug. The authors indicate that the results are equivocal. Two of the four patients improved with buspirone therapy. For these two children, improvement was noted in hyperactivity and aggression. No side effects were reported.

DEVELOPMENTAL PHARMACOKINETICS

(Pharmacokinetic data are not available in children or adolescents.)

Absorption: Buspirone is rapidly and completely absorbed. Buspirone peak blood levels occur in 60 to 90 minutes in adults. Administering buspirone with food slows the rate of absorption but increases the bioavailability.

Bioavailability: The oral bioavailability in adults is very low, about 4 percent (Kutcher et al., 1992).

Onset of action: In adults, the onset of action is within two to four weeks (Kutcher et al., 1992).

Duration of action: Unknown.

Half-life: In healthy adult volunteers the half-life of buspirone ranges from two to 11 hours (Kutcher et al., 1992).

Plasma levels: Plasma levels have not been evaluated in the pediatric population.

DOSAGE RANGES

Effective and safe doses of buspirone have not been evaluated for children or adolescents (*see* Studies of Buspirone Efficacy). Buspirone is chemically different from the benzodiazepines and will not block the withdrawal effects associated with the benzodiazepines.

ADVERSE EFFECTS REPORTED IN CHILDREN AND ADOLESCENTS

COMMON

Adverse effects reported in the open trial by Simeon (1993) include tiredness, nausea or stomach pains, and headaches. Common adverse effects of buspirone in the adult population include: nausea, dizziness, headache, insomnia, dysphoria, sedation, restlessness, chest pain, confusion, muscle weakness, numbness, tingling, pain, or weakness in hands or feet, uncontrolled movements of the body, sore throat, or fever.

LESS COMMON

Due to the lack of studies, there is a lack of information in this area. Until further information is available, practitioners are encouraged to monitor for the adverse effects that have been reported in adults (*see* Adverse Reactions/ Case Reports).

ALLERGIC REACTION: Unknown.

TOXICITY: Signs and symptoms of overdose in adults include severe dizziness, severe drowsiness, severe nausea or vomiting, and unusually small pupils.

ADVERSE REACTIONS/CASE REPORTS

Buspirone-Induced Psychosis

There is a case report of two children who developed psychotic symptoms while taking buspirone. Each of the children were treated for anxiety (Soni and Weintraub, 1992). The 12-year-old girl was treated with methylphenidate 15 mg three times daily for attention-deficit/hyperactivity disorder and pervasive developmental disorder. She was subsequently placed on buspirone 5 mg per day for four days and then increased to 5 mg two times daily. The patient developed loose associations, thought blocking, and odd behavior. Buspirone was discontinued, and the patient returned to baseline within 24 hours. The 11-year-old boy was treated with thioridazine 125 mg per day for post traumatic stress disorder. After the patient was placed on 5 mg of buspirone, he became more aggressive and the dose was increased to 5 mg two times daily. He subsequently developed inappropriate laughter and self-abuse, and he would stand still holding his hands in front of him while humming. Buspirone was discontinued and his symptoms resolved after three days. The authors suggest that the effects of buspirone are varied and that certain patients may be more vulnerable to buspirone-induced psychosis or aggression (Soni and Weintraub, 1992).

DRUG INTERACTIONS

DRUG	DRUGS	EFFECT
Buspirone	Digoxin	The effects of digoxin may be increased with buspirone therapy.

Buspirone	Monoamine oxidase inhibitors	Elevated blood pressure has occurred with the combination; it is not recommended.
Buspirone	Central nervous system depressants, including alcohol	The combination may result in increased sedative effect.
Buspirone	Haloperidol	The combination may result in elevated haloperidol serum levels.

MONITORING GUIDELINES

Baseline Assessment:

- History and physical, including weight and height of the patient.
- Blood pressure and pulse, white blood cell count with differential, electrolytes, urinalysis, and liver function tests. Other laboratory tests as indicated.

Time Pattern for Response:

- In adults, the onset of action occurs after two to four weeks of therapy. In the case studies reported of children, the effects of buspirone were observed with two to four days (*see* Studies of Buspirone Efficacy).

Follow-Up Assessment:

- Reassess the need for continued medication therapy.
- Monitor for adverse effects that are noted in the adult population.

Drug Discontinuation:

- In adults, abrupt withdrawal is not associated with rebound anxiety or withdrawal symptom.

SPECIAL INSTRUCTIONS FOR PARENTS/CARE GIVERS/ CHILDREN/ADOLESCENTS

- Buspirone may cause drowsiness or dizziness during the first few weeks. If this happens, the patient should not participate in activities that require alertness, such as riding a bike or driving a car.
- Inform the physician if any unusual reactions occur while taking buspirone.
- Store this medication and all medications away from the patient and other children and adolescents.
- Do not use alcohol or other depressants while taking buspirone.

PRODUCTS AVAILABLE

Buspirone is available as Buspar® and is marketed by Mead Johnson Pharmaceuticals.

Buspar® is marketed in a 5 mg ovoid-rectangular tablet that is white, scored, and imprinted with MJ, 5 mg, BuSpar. Buspar® is also marketed in a 10 mg ovoid-rectangular tablet that is white, scored, and imprinted with MJ, 10 mg, BuSpar.

COST

GENERIC NAME	TRADENAME	AWP*	AWP* per dose
Buspirone	Buspar® 5 mg	$55.59 for 100 tablets	$0.56 per tablet
	Buspar® 10 mg	$94.50 for 100 tablets	$0.95 per tablet

* AWP is the average wholesale price to the pharmacist that is listed in the *1994 Redbook* (Cardinale, 1994).

CARBAMAZEPINE

Carbamazepine

Tegretol® is marketed by Ciba Geigy Pharmaceuticals.

Epitol® is marketed by Lemmon Pharmaceuticals.

Carbamazepine is also available in generic form.

DSM-IV INDICATIONS

Aggression (???)

FDA: Approved for use as an anticonvulsant in children over six years of age (*PDR,* 1994).

USP: Appropriate studies have not been performed in children up to six years of age. However, behavioral changes are more likely to occur in children (*USPDI,* 1994).

CONTRAINDICATIONS: Hypersensitivity to carbamazepine or any drug with a tricyclic structure; history of previous bone marrow suppression; concurrent use with monoamine oxidase inhibitors (*see* Drug Interactions); hepatic or renal impairment; atrioventricular heart block; hyponatremia.

PHARMACOLOGY: Carbamazepine is a drug with numerous pharmacological effects including anticonvulsant, antiaggressive, and antimanic effects. Chemically, carbamazepine is a tricyclic structure, and resembles the antipsychotic chlorpromazine, and the tricyclic antidepressant imipramine. Carbamazepine blocks the release of norepinephrine, but inhibits the reuptake of norepinephrine from the presynaptic neuron. Carbamazepine does not appear to block dopamine receptors, but the pharmacological effects on dopamine are uncertain. The mechanism of action for carbamazepine's psychotropic effect may be related to the antikindling properties of the drug (Birkhimer, Curtis, and Jann, 1985). Kindling is a phenomenon of repeated subthreshold electrical stimulation that culminates in the development of major motor seizures or psychopathology. Carbamazepine is a very effective antikindling agent in the limbic and temporal lobe regions (Birkhimer, Curtis, and Jann, 1985).

STUDIES OF CARBAMAZEPINE EFFICACY

Aggression

Aggressive behavior is a nonspecific finding associated with a variety of psychiatric disorders. Kafantaris et al. (1992) reported an open pilot study using carbamazepine to treat aggressive and explosive children with conduct disorder. Ten seizure-free patients, with an age range of 5.25 to 10.92 years, were included. Patients were treated with three times daily administration of carbamazepine for three to five weeks, starting at carbamazepine 200 mg per day with increases to a maximum of 800 mg per day. Carbamazepine doses were titrated according to response, and ranged from 600 to 800 mg per day (mean 630 mg per day) with serum levels of 4.8 to 10.4 mcg/ml (mean of 6.2 mcg/ml). Carbamazepine reduced the target symptoms of fighting with peers, temper outbursts, and being a bully. On the Global Clinical Consensus Ratings, four patients were moderately and four patients were markedly improved. Adverse effects responded to dosage reduction and included fatigue, blurred vision, dizziness, diplopia, mild ataxia, mild dysarthria, headache, and lethargy. One patient developed loosening of associations and one patient's preexisting behavior become worse. Four patients had a reduction in white blood cells, but none were less than 4,000/mm^3. The authors indicate that further studies using double-blind, placebo-controlled conditions are warranted (Kafantaris et al., 1992).

DEVELOPMENTAL PHARMACOKINETICS

(The pharmacokinetics of carbamazepine in children and adolescents has not been adequately investigated.)

Absorption: The absorption of carbamazepine is slow with peak blood levels in three to six hours (Birkhimer, Curtis, and Jann,

1985). Meals may increase the absorption of carbamazepine. Carbamazepine tablets that are exposed to humidity will harden and have decreased absorption that may result in decreased blood levels and therapeutic effect.

Onset of action: Drowsiness may occur early in therapy, but a full therapeutic response in the treatment of aggression may take up to two weeks (Campbell, Gonzalez, and Silva, 1992).

Distribution: Carbamazepine is highly protein bound and alterations in protein binding as a result of drug interactions may increase the free or pharmacologically active fraction of carbamazepine. An increase in the free fraction may result in more therapeutic or toxic effects (Trimble, 1990).

Metabolism: Carbamazepine can induce its own metabolism. Maximum autoinduction of metabolism occurs at three to four weeks (Bertilsson et al., 1980). After two to six weeks of continuous therapy, dosage increases may be necessary to maintain therapeutic effects and blood levels. Carbamazepine is metabolized to an active metabolite, carbamazepine 10,11 epoxide (CBZ-E). CBZ-E has anticonvulsant and psychotropic effects (Birkhimer, Curtis, and Jann, 1985). Concurrent use of carbamazepine and other enzyme inducing drugs will increase the serum concentration and pharmacological activity of CBZ-E.

Duration of action: The duration of action is related to the half-life of carbamazepine.

Half-life: In a single-dose study of two children with epilepsy, the half-life of carbamazepine was 16.9 hours (Pynnonen, 1979). Autoinduction of metabolism (*see* Metabolism, above) is associated with a 40 to 50 percent reduction in half-life (Pynnonen, 1979). Increases in dose and decreases in the interval between doses may be required in order to maintain therapeutic blood levels. The Tegretol® product literature suggests administration of the drug three to four times per day in the treatment of seizures.

Serum levels: In the open study described above of ten children with conduct disorder, Kafantaris et al. (1992) reported therapeutic carbamazepine serum levels of 4.8 to 10.4 mcg/ml. In this study, a serum level of 12 mcg/ml was not exceeded. The dosage of carbamazepine should be titrated according to patient response within a serum concentration range of 4 to 12 mcg/ml. Carbamazepine serum levels should be monitored for the first two months to check for the effects of autoinduction. Further research is needed to substantiate that psychiatric disorders require carbamazepine serum levels in the upper range of 8 to 12 mcg/ml (Birkhimer, Curtis, and Jann, 1985). Due to the presence of the active metabolite, carbamazepine 10,11 epoxide, which is not routinely measured, toxicity may be observed with low or therapeutic serum levels of carbamazepine (Kafantaris et al., 1992). Carbamazepine 10,11 epoxide levels may be increased when carbamazepine is administered with enzyme inducers, including the neuroleptics, antidepressants, or barbiturates.

DOSAGE RANGES

Low doses (100 mg) should be initiated to avoid early side effects of nausea, ataxia, drowsiness and dizziness. The daily dose is gradually increased and adjusted according to patient response. Oral tablets should be administered at least three times per day to children. Adolescents may be dosed two to three times per day according to response. It is recommended to administer the suspension three to four times per day to avoid high peak and low trough serum levels. Carbamazepine can induce its own metabolism. Maximum autoinduction of metabolism occurs at three to four weeks. After two to four weeks of continuous therapy, dosage increases may be necessary to maintain therapeutic effects and blood levels. Carbamazepine is metabolized to an active metabolite, carbamazepine 10,11 epoxide (CBZ-E). Although not routinely measured, CBZ-E has anticonvulsant activity and possible psychotropic effects (Birkhimer, Curtis, and Jann, 1985).

> **Aggression:** Kafantaris et al. (1992) reported doses of 600 to 800 mg per day (mean of 630 mg per day) in the treatment of ten children with conduct disorder. Doses were administered in three divided doses and resulted in carbamazepine serum levels of 4.8 to 10.4 mcg/ml. Reduction in symptoms may be gradual, and two weeks of treatment

may be necessary before the therapeutic effect is observed (Campbell, Gonzalez, and Silva, 1992).

ADVERSE EFFECTS REPORTED IN CHILDREN AND ADOLESCENTS

COMMON

The adverse effects reported in children treated for aggression are fatigue, blurred vision, dizziness, diplopia, mild ataxia, mild dysarthria, headache, and lethargy (Kafantaris et al., 1992). Each of these side effects responded to dose reduction. Common adverse effects that are reported in children and adolescents treated with carbamazepine for seizures include: skin rash, nausea, drowsiness, incoordination, vertigo, ataxia, blurred vision, diplopia, tremor, headache, and slurred speech (Pellock, 1987). Mild skin rashes may progress to exfoliative, erythematous, and maculopapular dermatitis, requiring discontinuation of carbamazepine therapy. Reported adverse effects in children treated for conduct disorder and hyperactivity are irritability, aggressiveness, increased hyperactivity, emotional lability, angry outbursts, and insomnia (Evans, Clay, and Gualtieri, 1987). The central nervous system adverse effects may respond to dose reduction or discontinuation of carbamazepine.

LESS COMMON

Hyponatremia (Koivikko and Valikangas, 1983) syndrome of inappropriate anti-diuretic hormone, elevation of hepatic enzymes, granulomatous hepatitis, jaundice, heart block, dystonic reactions, chorea, dyskinesia, myoclonus, tics, loosening of associations (Kafantaris et al., 1992), behavioral problems, and mania have been reported (*see also* Adverse Reactions/Case Reports). Hematological abnormalities are associated with carbamazepine therapy including: thrombocytopenia, aplastic anemia, agranulocytosis, pancytopenia, and leukopenia. Due to the limited information in the area of adverse effects in children and adolescents, practitioners are encouraged to monitor for additional adverse effects that have been reported in adults.

ALLERGIC REACTION: Allergic skin rashes frequently occur and may require discontinuation of therapy.

TOXICITY: Nausea, vomiting, drowsiness, dizziness, ataxia, nystagmus, neuromuscular excitability, irregular breathing, tachycardia, hypotension, hypertension, urinary retention, oliguria, anuria, confusion, and seizures are signs and symptoms of carbamazepine toxicity (Trimble, 1990). Overdose of carbamazepine, a tricyclic structure, may result in mortality (Trimble, 1990).

ADVERSE REACTIONS/CASE REPORTS

Carbamazepine-Induced Mania

There are several case reports of carbamazepine inducing mania. Reiss and O'Donnell (1984) reported two ten-year-old boys who developed mania during therapy with carbamazepine. In both cases, the patient had a family history of bipolar disorder. The first case was treated for behavioral problems and complex partial seizures, and the second case was treated for fluctuating symptoms of depression and hypomania. In both cases, the mania developed within three weeks of initiation of carbamazepine therapy and abated upon discontinuation of carbamazepine. The second case had developed symptoms of mania during prior therapy with dextroamphetamine and imipramine. Pleak et al. (1988) reported the cases of two male patients, ages ten and 16 years old, who developed hypomania or mania during carbamazepine therapy. The 16-year-old was diagnosed with attention-deficit/hyperactivity disorder, conduct disorder, and rage outbursts. The ten year old was diagnosed with conduct disorder and aggressive outbursts. The carbamazepine induced mania or hypomania developed within one to three weeks following initiation of carbamazepine therapy.

Friedman et al. (1992) reported two male patients, ages 13 and 18 years old, with mental retardation that developed either hypomania or mania after treatment with carbamazepine. Both patients were treated with carbamazepine for self-injurious behavior, irritability, mood lability, or aggressiveness. Carbamazepine is chemically related to the tricyclic antidepressants, agents that may induce mania. Patients who have a family history of bipolar disorder or patients who have developed mania while taking other medications may be more susceptible to developing mania during carbamazepine therapy. Patients without a personal or family history of mania may also develop manic-like behavior. If manic-like symptoms develop, discontinuation of carbamazepine is indicated.

Carbamazepine-Induced Tics

Evans, Clay, and Gualtieri (1987) reported the case of a 7-year, 9-month-old Caucasian boy with hyperactivity, distractibility, short attention span, impulsiveness, aggressive behavior, destructiveness, and noncompliance. The patient responded to dextroamphetamine but developed tics that resolved as soon as the medication was discontinued. Due to electroencephalogram findings of paroxysmal sharp and slow wave activity, and independent right and left temporal sharp waves, a trial of carbamazepine was initiated. After six weeks on carbamazepine 700 mg per day, with a blood level of 4.6 mcg/ml (assumed to be incorrectly reported as ng/ml), the patient developed tic-like shoulder movements, phonic tics (throat clearing), and myoclonic movements of the entire body. The authors report that the movements continued for six weeks and subsided when carbamazepine was withdrawn (Evans, Clay, and Gualtieri, (1987). Kurlan et al. (1989) also reported a 13-year-old boy with Tourette's syndrome that developed worsening of tics on carbamazepine and phenytoin therapy.

Carbamazepine Associated with Behavioral Problems

Evans, Clay, and Gualtieri (1987) reported a ten-year-old Caucasian boy who had been treated with therapeutic levels of carbamazepine for seven years for unconfirmed reports of partial seizure activity. The patient had signs and symptoms of hyperactivity, inattention, impulsive behavior, emotional lability, irritability, and aggressive outbursts. The authors report that the patient's most troubling symptoms of irritability and aggressive outbursts subsided following discontinuation of carbamazepine. Residual problems of inattention and hyperactivity responded to methylphenidate. Friedman et al. (1992) reported an eight-year-old female patient with mental retardation that developed worsening of behavioral problems with carbamazepine. The patient developed increased self-injurious behaviors, irritability, hyperactivity, distractibility, and mood lability with carbamazepine therapy. The authors suggest that patients with mental retardation may be more susceptible to developing adverse effects, and if behavioral deterioration occurs, reevaluation of carbamazepine therapy is necessary. A complete baseline evaluation is necessary to determine the behavioral effects of carbamazepine.

DRUG INTERACTIONS

DRUG	DRUGS	EFFECT
Carbamazepine	Monoamine oxidase inhibitors	Concurrent use is contraindicated and may result in hyperpyretic crises, hypertensive crisis, convulsions, and death. A 14-day drug-free period is required between discontinuation of a monoamine oxidase inhibitor and initiation of carbamazepine.
Carbamazepine	Tricyclic antidepressants	Carbamazepine may enhance the metabolism of the tricyclic antidepressants and may require increases in the dose of the tricyclic antidepressant (Brown et al. 1990). Carbamazepine induced metabolism will increase the plasma levels of hydroxy metabolites of the tricyclic antidepressants. The hydroxy metabolites are pharma-

cologically active and possibly cardiotoxic but are not routinely measured or reported with tricyclic antidepressant plasma levels. Increased monitoring for cardiovascular effects is suggested when the combination is used (Baldessarini et al., 1988; De la Fuente, 1992).

Carbamazepine	Antipsychotics, stimulants, benzodiazepines	Carbamazepine may increase the metabolism and reduce the blood levels of these agents.
Carbamazepine	Cimetidine, erythromycin, propoxyphene, isoniazid, verapamil, diltiazem	Concurrent use may increase the serum levels of carbamazepine.
Carbamazepine	Acetaminophen, coumarin, doxycycline, theophylline, valproic acid, ethosuximide	Carbamazepine may decrease the blood levels or effectiveness of these agents.
Carbamazepine	Barbiturates, primidone	Concurrent use may increase the metabolism of carbamazepine and decrease serum levels.
Carbamazepine	Phenytoin	Concurrent administration may result in increased or decreased phenytoin levels and reduced carbamazepine levels. Therapeutic blood monitoring is indicated.
Carbamazepine	Lithium	Concurrent administration may result in enhanced therapeutic effect or neurotoxicity.
Carbamazepine	Desmopressin, vasopressin	Concurrent use may increase the antidiuretic effect that may result in lower sodium concentration and seizures.

Carbamazepine   Oral contraceptives   Concurrent use will decrease the effectiveness of the oral contraceptive, resulting in increased chance for pregnancy.

MONITORING GUIDELINES

Baseline Assessment:

- History and physical, including weight of the patient.
- Liver function tests, complete blood count with differential and platelet count, serum creatinine, BUN (Bun Urea Nitrogen), urine specific gravity, electrolytes, and electrocardiogram (Campbell, Gonzalez, and Silva, 1992).

Time Pattern for Response: In the treatment of aggression, the therapeutic effect occurs within two weeks (Campbell, Gonzalez, and Silva, 1992). A loss of therapeutic effect may occur between weeks two and six due to auto-induction of metabolism and a reduction in therapeutic serum levels. Dosage adjustments may be necessary. When carbamazepine is used in the treatment of aggression, the duration of therapy is six to 12 months, followed by gradual dose reduction (Trimble, 1990).

Follow-Up Assessment:

- A complete blood count (CBC) with differential and platelet count should be obtained according to patient status. Sobotka, Alexander, and Cook (1990) recommend that if the pretreatment or baseline CBC with differential and platelet counts are in the middle to upper normal range, no further laboratory checks are necessary unless signs or symptoms of possible hematological abnormalities are observed. If the baseline blood indices are in the low normal or below-normal range, these patients should have repeat monitoring every two weeks for the first one to three months of treatment. If the white blood cell count is less than 3,000/mm^3 or a neutrophil count is less than 1,000/mm^3 the dose of carbamazepine should be reduced or discontinued depending upon the patient's status (Sobotka, Alexander, and Cook, 1990). Aplastic anemia, agranulocytosis, and thrombocytopenia may develop within one to two days and may not be detected with weekly blood monitoring. All patients should be informed to monitor for signs and symptoms of fever, fatigue, infections, lymphadenopathy, bruising, or bleeding through mucous membranes, and to report the findings immediately to the physician (Sobotka, Alexander, and Cook, 1990).

- Serum carbamazepine levels should be obtained during dosage titration or if there is a deterioration in response. The autoinduction of metabolism will reduce the serum concentration of carbamazepine, and symptoms of the disorder may reappear. Maximal enzyme induction may occur up to six weeks after initiation of therapy and dosage adjustments are necessary to maintain therapeutic response.
- Liver function tests should be obtained according to patient status. Patients should be informed to monitor for malaise, anorexia, lethargy, stomach fullness, yellowing of skin and eyes, dark urine, pale stools, and fluid retention, and to report to the physician.
- Monitor for adverse central nervous system effects including worsening of behavior. Dosage reduction or discontinuation of carbamazepine may be indicated.

Drug Discontinuation:

- Gradual withdrawal is indicated and withdrawal seizures may occur in patients with no prior history of seizures. The schedule of dosage reduction depends on the dose, the duration of therapy, and the reason for discontinuation. Discontinuation of carbamazepine may result in increased blood levels of concurrently administered medications (e.g., theophylline) resulting in toxicity; therefore, drug interactions need to be assessed.

SPECIAL INSTRUCTIONS FOR PARENTS/CARE GIVERS/ CHILDREN/ADOLESCENTS

- Carbamazepine may cause drowsiness, dizziness, or clumsiness during the first few weeks. If this happens, the patient should not participate in activities that require alertness, such as riding a bike or driving a car.
- Take this medication with food to avoid stomach upset.
- If the patient develops a fever, sore throat, ulcers in the mouth, bruising, or bleeding, stop the medication and contact the physician immediately.
- If the patient develops tiredness, loss of appetite, lack of energy, stomach fullness, yellowing of skin and eyes, dark urine, pale stools, swelling of the legs or feet, increased or decreased urination, vomiting, rash, increased behavioral problems, or any other unusual reaction, contact the physician as soon as possible.
- This medication may make your skin more sensitive to sunburn. Be sure to use a sunscreen lotion and wear protective clothing when outside.
- Do not stop taking carbamazepine without checking with your physician. The physician will want to decrease the dosage of carbamazepine slowly before stopping completely.
- Blood tests are needed prior to starting carbamazepine and according to the patient's status. Blood tests are needed to determine the amount of carbamazepine in the blood and to watch for possible side effects.
- Be sure to store this product in a cool, dry place, and away from showers, bathrooms, and humidifiers. Humidity may harden the tablets and reduce the effectiveness of the medication. Be sure to shake the suspension before using.
- Be sure to tell all physicians, pharmacists, and dentists that this medication is being taken.
- Do not take any other medication without checking with your physician or pharmacist.

- Store this medication and all medications away from the patient and other children and adolescents.
- Avoid the use of alcoholic beverages during therapy with this medication.

PRODUCTS AVAILABLE

Carbamazepine is available as Tegretol® from Ciba Geigy Pharmaceuticals and as Epitol® from Lemmon Pharmaceuticals. Carbamazepine is also available in generic form.

Epitol® is marketed in a 200 mg white, scored, round, convex tablet imprinted with Epitol 93,93, T, 109.

Tegretol® is marketed in a 100 mg chewable, scored, red speckled and pink, round tablet imprinted with Tegretol 52. Tegretol® is also marketed in a 200 mg scored, pink, capsule-shaped, tablet imprinted with Tegretol 27. Tegretol® suspension is yellow-orange, citrus-vanilla flavored and contains carbamazepine 100 mg per 5 ml.

COST

GENERIC NAME	TRADENAME	AWP*	AWP* per dose
Carbamazepine 200 mg		$17.28 for 100 tablets	$0.18 per tablet
Carbamazepine 100 mg chewable		$18.67 for 100 tablets	$0.19 per tablet
Carbamazepine	Epitol® 200 mg	$24.00 for 100 tablets	$0.24 per tablet
	Tegretol® 200 mg	$34.66 for 100 tablets	$0.35 per tablet
	Tegretol® 100 mg chewable	$18.00 for 100 tablets	$0.18 per tablet
	Tegretol® 100 mg per 5 ml suspension	$24.80 for 500 ml	$0.25 per 5 ml

* AWP is the average wholesale price to the pharmacist that is listed in the *1994 Redbook* (Cardinale, 1994).

CLONIDINE

Clonidine hydrochloride

Catapres® is marketed by Boehringer Ingelheim.

Clonidine is also available in generic form.

DSM-IV INDICATIONS

Attention-Deficit/Hyperactivity Disorder (??)

Gilles de la Tourette's syndrome (??)

Autism (???)

Aggression (???)

> FDA: Safety and efficacy have not been established in the pediatric population (*PDR*, 1994).
>
> USP: Indications include Gilles de la Tourette's syndrome but specify that appropriate studies in pediatrics have not been done (*USPDI*, 1994).

CONTRAINDICATIONS: Hypersensitivity to clonidine; cardiovascular disease or mental depression. For the transdermal product, skin irritation or disease is a contraindication.

PHARMACOLOGY: Clonidine hydrochloride is an alpha adrenergic agonist. The antihypertensive effect of clonidine is thought to be due to the activation of the autoinhibitory presynaptic alpha receptors that reduce the endogenous release of norepinephrine. The reduction of norepinephrine leads to decreased sympathetic outflow to the heart, kidneys, and peripheral vasculature, and results in decreased peripheral vascular resistance, decreased systolic and diastolic blood pressure, and decreased heart rate. In addition, clonidine reduces the firing rate of the locus coeruleus and decreases excessive arousal.

Clonidine is a potent short-term stimulator of growth hormone secretion. As such, it has been investigated in the treatment of constitutional growth delay (CGD). Children with CGD have normal growth hormone releasing hormone and growth hormone reserves but have a transient defect in growth hormone release. The results of two 12-month placebo-controlled, double-blind, randomized, crossover studies indicate a lack of growth response to clonidine treatment (Pescovitz and Tan, 1988; Allen, 1993). Currently, the use of clonidine to treat children with CGD is not recommended because they will reach normal adult height eventually without therapy (Toy and Middleton, 1991), and clonidine is not without risk to the patient. In addition, alpha-2 adrenergic agonists may down-regulate adrenergic receptors when administered chronically (greater than six months). Therefore, the effects of clonidine on growth acceleration appear to be transient.

STUDIES OF CLONIDINE EFFICACY

Aggression

Kemph et al. (1993) conducted a preliminary open outpatient investigation of 17 highly aggressive children (aged five to 15 years) with conduct/oppositional disorder. Participants were selected to participate based on their severely aggressive behavior relating to people and property, and their failure to respond to behavioral management. Oral clonidine was initiated at 0.05 mg/ day for two days, then increased to 0.05 mg twice a day for two days, and finally increased to 0.05 mg three times daily if tolerated. Doses were adjusted according to levels of drowsiness. Assessments of the participants were conducted at baseline and at one month. At one month, three patients were no longer aggressive, nine patients were considered mildly aggressive, and three were considered moderate to severely aggressive. One patient was non-compliant and was unchanged from baseline, and one patient was lost to follow-up. Clonidine oral doses ranged from 0.15 to 0.4 mg per day. Drowsiness was the most common adverse effect and there was no significant change in blood pressure or untoward cardiovascular changes in this study group. This open trial is very encouraging considering the violent nature of the study participants. Further placebo-controlled investigations of clonidine in the treatment of aggression are suggested.

Attention-Deficit Disorder with Hyperactivity (ADDH)

Hunt, Minderaa, and Cohen (1985) and Hunt (1987) performed two separate trials to determine the effect of clonidine in the treatment of ADDH. The first trial (Hunt, Minderaa, and Cohen, 1985) was placebo-controlled and double-blind. Two girls and eight boys aged 11.6 ± 0.54 years received 0.004 to 0.005 mg/kg/day of oral clonidine for eight consecutive weeks. In order to participate in the study each child fulfilled the DSM-III diagnostic criteria for attention-deficit disorder with hyperactivity, and a score of at least 2.0 standard deviations above normal on the Hyperactivity Index of the Conners' scales as rated by either parent or teacher. Parents and teachers rated each child every two weeks using the Conners' Parent Behavior Rating and the Teachers Behavior Rating scales, respectively. Parents and children were interviewed on videotape on a monthly basis. Parents reported a 25 to 50 percent improvement during clonidine treatment in seven children. Three of the children, including both girls, showed no overall change according to their parents. Teachers' ratings were obtained for eight of the ten children. The teachers ratings indicated improvement of 25 to 75 percent in five of the eight children. Clinicians rated improvement of 25 to 75 percent in eight of the children.

In a second study (Hunt, 1987), the effectiveness of oral and transdermal clonidine were compared with placebo and methylphenidate. Seven boys and one girl (age range 6.7 to 14.4 years) were included in this open, pilot study. Children fulfilled the DSM-III criteria for ADDH. Each child was randomly treated with placebo, methylphenidate low dose (0.3 mg/kg/day) and high dose (0.6 mg/kg/day) for one week. Clonidine was then initiated and titrated to 0.005 mg/kg/day for eight weeks. Responders to oral clonidine were then switched to the transdermal product, at an equivalent dose. Parents and teachers reported that clonidine was more effective than placebo and equally effective as methylphenidate. There was minimal difference between the oral and transdermal routes of administration of clonidine.

To establish the efficacy of clonidine in the treatment of Attention-Deficit/Hyperactivity Disorder (ADHD) (DSM-IV criteria), larger controlled studies need to be conducted. Hunt, Capper, and

O'Connell (1990) suggest that clonidine appears more effective than stimulants in reducing high levels of motor activity and subjective arousal. Clonidine may be more effective for children with ADHD and comorbid tic disorders, extreme overactivity, oppositional disorder, conduct disorder, poor response to stimulants, or hyperarousal (Hunt, Capper, and O'Connell, 1990). Rubenstein, Silver, and Licamele (1994) in a case report of a child with ADHD, suggest that the sedative effects of clonidine may be useful in treating stimulant induced insomnia and to cover the effects of the stimulant wearing off.

Attention-Deficit/Hyperactivity Disorder (ADHD) with Comorbid Tic Disorder

Steingard et al. (1993) retrospectively studied the charts of 54 children with ADHD with or without a comorbid tic disorder. The assessment was determined from clinic notes, and parent and teacher reports. The study suggests that children with ADHD and comorbid tic disorder had a more positive behavioral response to clonidine than children with ADHD without a tic disorder. Patients with comorbid tic disorders experienced a moderate reduction in the frequency of their tics. The findings were consistent regardless of previous stimulant or antidepressant response. The dosages of clonidine administered ranged from 0.025 to 0.6 mg/day with a mean dose of 0.2 mg/day. When each patient was assessed and over what period of time were not described. The authors acknowledge the uncontrolled design of their study including the unstructured visit schedules, but suggest future controlled studies.

Autism

One open study and two double-blind preliminary studies have been conducted in children with autism. An open study by Ghaziuddin, Tsai, and Ghaziuddin (1992) studied seven patients (five males, two females, mean age 6.5 ± 1.4 years) with DSM-III-R autistic disorder who also had symptoms of hyperactivity, impulsivity, and impairment of attention. Six of the seven children had mental retardation ranging from moderate to severe. Patients achieved maintenance doses in six to eight weeks with clinical improvement in the dosing range of 0.15 to 0.20 mg/day. Five of the seven patients were rated with moderate to marked improvement on the Conners' ten-item parent-teacher scale, parent and teacher reports, and clinical observation. One patient had slight improvement and one patient had no improvement. Sedation was the most common adverse effect. The authors suggest that clonidine may be beneficial for patients with autism and hyperactivity, attentional problems, and impulsivity.

Jaselskis et al. (1992) studied eight male children (ages 8.1 ± 2.8 years) in a double-blind crossover study of oral clonidine. Children were included in the study if they had autistic disorder diagnosed by DSM-III-R criteria and inattention, impulsivity, and hyperactivity. Subjects included had not responded to neuroleptics, methylphenidate, or desipramine. Full scale IQs ranged from 30 to 75 (59 ± 16) indicating various degrees of mental retardation. The patients were randomly assigned to begin clonidine or placebo. Each patient was drug free for four weeks prior to the study. Clonidine or placebo was titrated up over two weeks to a dose of 0.004 to 0.010 mg/kg/day administered in three divided doses daily. Dosages were titrated downward for significant adverse effects under double-blind conditions. Each phase of the crossover lasted six weeks followed by tapering over one week and then crossover to the second phase. Parents and teachers rated the child on a weekly basis for efficacy and adverse effects. For clinician ratings, three 15-minute videotape sessions were conducted, at baseline and after each phase of the study.

The parent ratings on the Conners Parent-Teacher Questionnaire showed a statistically significant improvement with clonidine therapy. Teacher ratings of irritability, hyperactivity, stereotypy, and inappropriate speech were statistically improved also. Even though the parent and teacher ratings reached statistical significance, clinically there was only modest improvement. In addition, there was no significant improvement in attention and hyperactivity. Parents and teachers indicated a significant increase in drowsiness and decreased activity on clonidine. The clinician ratings did not show significant differences between clonidine and placebo. After the study, six of the eight patients continued on clonidine in an open fashion. Four of the six patients developed tolerance to the therapeutic effect of clonidine after six to eight weeks of therapy. Higher doses of clonidine led to hypotension, drowsiness, and increased irritability; therefore, clonidine was subsequently discontinued. Two of the patients continued on clonidine for one year after the study without signs of tolerance.

Fankhauser et al. (1992) studied the use of transdermal clonidine in seven children and two adults with autism. Subjects were randomly assigned to initially receive either clonidine (approximately 0.005 mg/kg/day) or placebo by a weekly transdermal patch. Each phase of the crossover trial was four weeks with a two-week washout period between treatment phases. Subjects were evaluated every two weeks by clinicians and every week by parents. The authors note that clonidine therapy resulted in significantly fewer sensory responses (e.g., not agitated by noises and new activities, less whirling/spinning of objects, less repetitive behaviors and vocalizations), less affectual reactions (e.g., fewer abrupt affect changes and temper outbursts), and improved social relationships to people (e.g., appropriate responses to interactions and activities, initiating appropriate interactions, less isolation or ignoring interaction attempt, and less disruptive behavior). Clinicians and parents felt that for the majority of subjects, clonidine produced a calming or anti-anxiety effect that reduced inattention and repetitive behaviors and improved their ability to initiate and respond to social interactions. The authors note that clonidine therapy was associated with fatigue and sedation during the first two weeks, but was considered minimal by week four (Fankhauser et al., 1992).

Gilles de la Tourette's Syndrome

The efficacy of clonidine in Tourette's disorder is controversial. The initial open or single blind studies were promising (Cohen et al., 1980; Borison et al., 1983; Leckman et al., 1985; Singer, Gammon, and Quaskey, 1985-86). In addition, a double-blind 12-week study of 40 subjects (31 subjects were under 18 years of age) showed that clonidine was more efficacious than placebo on a global scale and specifically for motor tics. Parents rated clonidine over placebo for symptoms of impulsivity and hyperactivity; however, clinician rating showed little to no improvement (Leckman et al., 1991). Investigators (Cohen et al., 1980; Leckman et al., 1985) have suggested that the behavioral manifestations of Tourette's syndrome, such as compulsive acts or hyperactivity, are more responsive to clonidine, with little or no change in the frequency of vocal or motor tics.

In contrast, Shapiro, Shapiro, and Eisenkraft (1983) found in an open trial comparing neuroleptics to clonidine that neuroleptics were more effective than clonidine across a broad spectrum of Tourette's symptoms. A double-blind, placebo-controlled study by Goetz et al. (1987) indicates that clonidine did not reduce motor tics, vocalizations, or behavioral manifestations. This study was well controlled with blinded reviewers and videotaped examinations. Comparisons were made between children and adults, concurrent neuroleptic use or not, high dose (0.015 mg/kg/day) and low dose (0.0075 mg/kg/day) clonidine, and twice a day versus three times a day dosing. This investigation included 24 children and six adults. Thirteen patients felt that they had improved globally on clonidine, whereas nine felt that they had improved globally on placebo.

The issue of drug therapy for Tourette's syndrome is controversial. The decision is whether to begin neuroleptic treatment, which is more effective but carries the risk of tardive dyskinesia and other adverse effects, or to give a trial of clonidine to determine response. Results from investigations indicate that the efficacy of clonidine for Tourette's varies from no improvement to improvement on some measurements, to improvement on all symptoms. Investigators have suggested that clonidine is effective on a short-term basis while others suggest that benefit develops gradually. To add to the controversy, Comings et al. (1990) suggest that a different route of administration of clonidine (transdermal) is more efficacious than the oral route, especially for some patients. Considering the limited number of investigations and study participants, it is possible that a subpopulation of patients with Tourette's syndrome will respond to clonidine.

DEVELOPMENTAL PHARMACOKINETICS

Absorption:

Oral route: Clonidine is well absorbed from the gastrointestinal tract.

Transdermal route: Transdermal absorption in children has not been studied. For dosing considerations, children may absorb topically applied drugs more completely than adults. In addition, children have a greater surface area relative to total body mass than adults (Shear and Raddle, 1993). There are differences in absorption depending upon the site of application. In adults, the absorption from the upper outer arm or the torso is comparable, but the absorption from the thigh is decreased.

Onset of action: Sedation occurs early in therapy; therapeutic response may take two to eight weeks.

Time to peak effect: Sedation peaks at 30 to 90 minutes post oral administration (Hunt, Capper, and O'Connel, 1990).

Duration of action:

Oral route: Behavioral effects last three to six hours (Hunt, Capper, and O'Connell, 1990).

Transdermal: The patch is designed to last seven days, however, Hunt (1987) reported that for the treatment of ADHD, the effects may last only for five days.

Half-life: In a study of seven children, the half-life ranged from 6.4 to 18.6 hours (Leckman et al., 1986).

Plasma levels: Plasma levels of clonidine have been reported in a study of seven children. Trough levels range from 0.22 to 0.57 ng/nl, 12 hours after the dose (Leckman et al., 1986). Therapeutic blood levels have not been studied in children and are listed for informational purposes only.

DOSAGE RANGES

Aggression: For patients five to 15 years of age, Kemph et al. (1993) utilized initial oral doses of 0.05 mg/day and titrated up by 0.05 mg/day every two days according to sedation. Doses at one month ranged from 0.15 to 0.4 mg/day and were administered in divided doses three times daily.

Attention-Deficit/Hyperactivity Disorder:

Oral: Doses of 0.003 to 0.005 mg/kg/day have been studied (Hunt, Minderaa, and Cohen, 1985; Hunt, 1987). Hunt, Capper, and O'Connell (1990) report that the median dose for an eight- to 12-year-old is 0.25 to 0.3 mg/day and for adolescents is it 0.3 to 0.4 mg/day.

Transdermal: Oral doses up to 0.005 mg/kg/day were switched to the transdermal product, at an equivalent dose (Hunt, 1987). Hunt (1987) reported that for the treatment of ADHD, the effects may last only five days. The transdermal patch is designed for once a week dosing in adults.

Autism:

Oral: Jaselskis et al. (1992) studied oral clonidine doses of 0.004 to 0.010 mg/kg/day divided into three daily doses.

Transdermal: Fankhauser et al. (1992) studied transdermal clonidine doses of 0.005 mg/kg/day.

Tourette's Syndrome:

Oral: Doses vary across studies with a range of 0.003 to 0.015 mg/kg/day. The usual starting dose is 0.05 mg daily and then increased by 0.05 mg per day, titrated to the amount of sedation. Doses are administered on a two to three times daily dosing regimen.

Transdermal: Comings et al. (1990) recommend the clonidine patch over oral dosage forms. The starting dose is one-fourth of a 0.1 mg transdermal patch applied every week, then gradually inch over weeks to months as needed. Comings et al. suggest that the patch can be effective when oral doses are not.

ADVERSE EFFECTS REPORTED IN CHILDREN AND ADOLESCENTS

COMMON

Sedation (problematic during the first two to four weeks of therapy), dry mouth, restlessness, hypotension, postural hypotension, headache, dizziness, stomachache, nausea, and vomiting. Depression may occur but is found more commonly in patients with a predisposition to depressive disorders. Upon abrupt withdrawal, elevations in systolic and diastolic blood pressure and pulse may occur. For the transdermal product the adverse effects are the same with the addition of skin irritation which occurs in 20 to 30 percent of patch users. Skin irritation can be minimized by moving the patch to a different area on the body every few days.

LESS COMMON

Constipation, changes in appetite, sodium and water retention, Raynaud's phenomena (*see also* Adverse Reactions/Case Reports)

ALLERGIC REACTION: The manufacturer indicates that patients who have developed a localized skin rash to the transdermal product may, if switched to the oral product, develop a generalized skin rash. In addition, patients who develop a generalized skin rash to the transdermal product may develop a similar reaction if switched to the oral product. Hunt, Capper, and O'Connell (1990) suggest that this finding is uncommon in their clinical practice.

TOXICITY: The manufacturer indicates that the signs and symptoms of clonidine overdose include: hypotension, bradycardia, lethargy, irritability, weakness, somnolence, diminished or absent reflexes, miosis, vomiting, and hypoventilation. Large overdoses are associated with arrhythmias, apnea, seizures, and transient hypertension. (*See also* Adverse Reactions/Case Reports.)

ADVERSE REACTIONS/CASE REPORTS

Clonidine Toxicity

There are four case reports of clonidine toxicity resulting from the accidental application or ingestion of the transdermal patch by infants or toddlers (Harris, 1990; 1991). The patches were either inadvertently removed from the care givers skin or taken out of the garbage by the child. The signs and symptoms reported include irritability, anorexia, increased fluid intake and urine output, progressive lethargy, bradycardia, miosis, and gasping respirations. The author notes the attraction of children to bandages or stickers and the likelihood of toxicity from the patch. The patch contains an excess amount of drug (approximately three times the weekly dose) to maintain the concentration gradient for drug delivery. Ingestion of the patch is likely to result in quick onset of toxicity due to the absorption of clonidine through the mucous membranes. Refer to Instructions for Parents/Care Givers/Children/Adolescents for comments on safe keeping and disposal of the patch.

Hyperglycemia Associated with Clonidine

Mimouni-Bloch and Mimouni (1993) reported a case study of a 9.5-year-old girl with type I diabetes mellitus. The patient was stabilized on 4 units of insulin per day for six months. She subsequently developed tics, and Tourette's syndrome was diagnosed and treated with 0.050 mg of clonidine per day. The tics disappeared within a few days but the patient developed hyperglycemia requiring insulin doses up to 56 units per day. Following discontinuation of clonidine the patient developed hypoglycemia and the insulin dose was decreased to 6 units per day.

Cardiac Dysrhythmia Associated with Clonidine

Dawson et al. (1989) published a case report of a ten-year-old boy who was treated with clonidine for intermittent explosive disorder. The patient had been receiving propranolol 100 mg three times daily prior to the clonidine. While on propranolol the patient had a normal electrocardiogram (ECG) with sinus bradycardia (54 beats/ minute). The patient was tapered off of the propranolol over eight days and was off of propranolol one day prior to clonidine initiation. Clonidine was initiated at 0.05 mg for two doses. The patient's pulse was slow and irregular, blood pressure was normal and unchanged from previous readings. The patient's ECG showed marked sinus dysrhythmia, bradycardia (46 beats/minute), first-degree heart block, and several nonconducted P waves. Clonidine was discontinued and the ECG was normal the following day (heart rate 64 beats/minute).

Pain Associated with Clonidine

Kerbeshian and Burd (1987) reported a 14-year-old female who was prescribed clonidine for Tourette's syndrome. The patient developed multifocal joint pain, and sharp and persistent bilateral flank pain after taking clonidine 0.05 mg. The pain started within 15 minutes of taking a dose and lasted approximately 45 minutes. Dosage reductions decreased the pain and with a dose of 0.0125 mg/day the pain persisted for less than 15 minutes. The patient also reported "hyped" thinking when taking clonidine which made it difficult for her to complete her school work. The clonidine was discontinued, and haloperidol was initiated with a good response.

Transient Exacerbation of Tics Associated with Clonidine

Huk (1989) reported an 11-year-old boy with a history of severe behavioral problems diagnosed with Tourette's syndrome. The patient was started on 0.05 mg/day of clonidine that was titrated to 0.1 mg two times daily over a two-week period of time. It was retrospectively observed that when the patient was receiving the intermediate dose of clonidine 0.15 mg per day there was an exacerbation of the tics. The subsequent to the final dose abated the tics. Follow-up in six months resulted in continued improvement on the final dose.

Precocious Puberty Associated with Clonidine

Levin, Burton-Teston, and Murphy (1993) reported two seven-year-old girls who were treated with clonidine for hyperactivity and aggressive behavior. Both patients had received other psychotropic agents prior to clonidine therapy; however, both patients were taking clonidine 0.2 to 0.3 mg/day alone when they developed early pubertal signs. The progression of puberty stopped upon discontinuation of clonidine. The patients were monitored for one year following the discontinuation of clonidine. Precocious puberty is defined in females as the presence of breasts or pubic hair before the age nine years or menses before the age of ten. Confirmatory laboratory tests such as gonadotropin levels or bone X-rays were not obtained due to family financial restraints, therefore actual puberty or other medical conditions were not definitively ruled out. The authors considered various factors that could have contributed to the early puberty, but concluded that the abrupt halting of the progression of puberty after discontinuing the clonidine made the other factors less likely. The authors encourage clinicians to monitor for physical signs of precocious puberty in patients treated with clonidine.

DRUG INTERACTIONS

DRUG	DRUGS	EFFECT
Clonidine	Anticholinergic agents	Enhanced anticholinergic effect.
Clonidine	Anti-hypertensive agents	Increased hypotensive effect.
Clonidine	Beta-Blockers	Concurrent use of a beta-blocking drug during clonidine withdrawal may exacerbate the rebound hypertension. It is recommended that the beta-blocker be discontinued several days prior to discontinuation of clonidine.
Clonidine	CNS Depressants	Enhanced CNS depressant effect.
Clonidine	Fenfluramine	Increased hypotensive effect of clonidine.
Clonidine	Tricyclic antidepressants, sympathomimetics, anti-inflammatory agents	Reduced hypotensive effect of clonidine for treating hypertension.

MONITORING GUIDELINES

Baseline Assessment:

- History and physical, including weight of the patient.
- Blood pressure and pulse, electrocardiogram, electrolytes (serum sodium, glucose), and liver function tests. Other laboratory tests as indicated.
- Determine the family or individual history of diabetes mellitus. If positive, then assess the risk to benefit ratio for the possibility of clonidine precipitating diabetes mellitus (Leckman et al., 1985).

Time Pattern for Response: Sedation routinely occurs during the initial dosage titration and tolerance subsequently develops. Therapeutic effect occurs in two to eight weeks.

Follow-Up Assessment:

- Blood pressure and pulse should routinely be obtained during dose titration and during follow-up.
- Monitor for sedation during the dose titration period and during follow-up.
- Monitor body weight and appetite changes on a monthly basis.
- Monitor for continued effect: tolerance to the effect of clonidine has been reported after several months of therapy (Cohen et al., 1980).
- Monitor for symptoms of diabetes mellitus. If positive, fasting blood glucose and two-hour postprandial glucose specimens are recommended (Leckman et al., 1985)
- Laboratory work-up: According to patient status.

Drug Discontinuation:

- Abrupt withdrawal is not recommended. Elevation in systolic and diastolic blood pressure and pulse is reported within 24 to 72 hours after abrupt discontinuation in children (Leckman et al., 1985) and exacerbation of tics has been reported. Tic exacerbation will not be immediately alleviated by restarting clonidine. Patients may require

two to 16 weeks of clonidine therapy before tics abate
(Leckman et al., 1986).
• Withdrawal over seven days is recommended (Leckman
et al., 1983).

SPECIAL INSTRUCTIONS FOR PARENTS/CARE GIVERS/ CHILDREN/ADOLESCENTS

• Clonidine may cause drowsiness during the first few weeks.
If this happens, the child should not participate in activities
that require alertness, such as riding a bike or driving a car.
• Do not use any other medications without consulting your
physician or pharmacist.
• Do not stop taking or giving clonidine suddenly, without
checking with your physician. Usually, the medication is decreased slowly over several days.
• If a dose is missed, give it or take it as soon as possible, then
go back to the regular dosing schedule. Do not double dose.
If several doses are missed, contact your physician.
• Store this medication and all medications away from the patient and other children and adolescents.

TRANSDERMAL PATCHES (Harris, 1990):

– Keep the unused product out of the reach of children.
– Place the patch on parts of the body inaccessible to the child
or other children.
– The patch should be placed on a part of the body that is
without hair, scars, or irritation.
– If mild skin irritation occurs around the patch, move it to a
new site. Apply each new patch to a different site.
– The patch should stay in place during showers, bathing, or
swimming; however, if it becomes loose, cover it with the
extra adhesive covering. The patch may need to be replaced
after extended swimming or in humid weather.
– Even after use, the patch contains a significant amount of
active drug.
– Keep track of each patch and dispose of it by folding the
sticky sides together and placing the patch in a garbage can
inaccessible to children.

PRODUCTS AVAILABLE

Clonidine hydrochloride is available as Catapres® from Boehringer Ingelheim and is available as a generic product.

Catapres® is marketed in 0.1 mg (tan, BI 6), 0.2 mg (orange, BI 7), 0.3 mg (peach, BI 11) oval shaped, single scored tablets. Generic products are available in the same dosage strengths.

Catapres® is also available in a transdermal therapeutic system. Catapres-TTS-1®, Catapres-TTS-2® and Catapres-TTS-3® deliver 0.1 mg, 0.2 mg, and 0.3 mg per day respectively over a one-week period. Each of the Catapres-TTS® patches is cut from a large sheet of the product according to the designated surface area. The Catapres-TTS-3® contains three times more drug than the Catapres-TTS-1®. A lack of damage to the integrity of the rate controlling membrane cannot be totally assured when cutting a patch; therefore, cutting of the transdermal patch is not recommended by the manufacturer (Boehringer Ingelheim, personal communication).

Clonidine is available as a generic product in 0.1 mg, 0.2 mg, and 0.3 mg tablets.

COST

GENERIC NAME	TRADENAME	AWP*	AWP* per dose
Clonidine 0.1 mg		$6.00 for 100 tablets	$0.06 per tablet
Clonidine 0.2 mg		$8.50 for 100 tablets	$0.09 per tablet
Clonidine 0.3 mg		$10.50 for 100 tablets	$0.11 per tablet
Clonidine	Catapres® 0.1 mg	$54.22 for 100 tablets	$0.55 per tablet
	Catapres® 0.2 mg	$82.87 for 100 tablets	$0.83 per tablet
	Catapres® 0.3 mg	$104.12 for 100 tablets	$1.05 per tablet
	Catapres-TTS-1®	$87.58/12 patches	$7.29 per patch
	Catapres-TTS-2®	$147.43/12 patches	$12.29 per patch
	Catapres-TTS-3®	$68.10/4 patches	$ 17.02 per patch

* AWP is the average wholesale price to the pharmacist that is listed in the *1994 Redbook* (Cardinale, 1994).

DESMOPRESSIN

Desmopressin acetate

DDAVP® is marketed by Rhone-Poulenc Rorer.

DSM-IV INDICATIONS

Primary Nocturnal Enuresis

FDA: Safe and moderately effective in children six years and older with severe nocturnal enuresis. Adequately controlled studies beyond four to eight weeks have not been conducted.

USP: Accepted therapy for primary nocturnal enuresis.

CONTRAINDICATIONS: Known hypersensitivity to DDAVP® nasal spray.

PHARMACOLOGY: Desmopressin acetate is a synthetic analogue of the natural anti-diuretic hormone 8-arginine vasopressin. Desmopressin is chemically defined as 1-(3-mercaptopropionic acid)-8-D-arginine vasopressin monoacetate trihydrate. The structural modification of 8-arginine vasopressin to desmopressin acetate increases the antidiuretic effect, decreases the vasopressor action and the effect on visceral smooth muscle at low doses. Desmopressin increases water reabsorption in the kidney by increasing the cellular permeability of the collecting ducts, resulting in increased urine osmolality and decreased urine output.

Currently, there is no animal data to suggest that desmopressin therapy exerts a negative feedback effect on the hypothalamic-neurohypophyseal axis that would result in decreased endogenous vasopressin secretion (Hjalmas and Bengtsson, 1993). Knudsen et al. (1991) reported eight patients, ages 11 to 24 years, who were given desmopressin for 24 weeks. There was no difference in baseline and post-therapy vasopressin plasma concentrations suggesting that desmopressin does not influence endogenous vasopressin production. Rew and Rundle (1989) reported on a group of seven patients aged ten to 26 years who received desmopressin therapy for an average of 13 months (range four to 24 months). A follow-up assessment of blood count, blood urea, electrolytes, creatinine, liver function tests, and a static endocrine profile of thyroxine, luteinizing hormone, follicle stimulating hormone, and prolactin were normal in all patients. Each patient omitted desmopressin therapy for one day to undergo a standardized water deprivation test. The results indicated that the body could still concentrate the urine, even after months of desmopressin therapy. These results suggest that desmopressin does not alter normal development.

STUDIES OF DESMOPRESSIN EFFICACY

Primary Nocturnal Enuresis

The treatment of choice for primary nocturnal enuresis is the enuresis alarm, which is the only therapy proven to provide a lasting cure.

One of the many theories about the pathogenesis of nocturnal enuresis is that patients with enuresis lack the normal nocturnal rise in the secretion of endogenous arginine vasopressin (Norgaard, Ritting, and Djurhuus, 1989). Therefore, nocturnal enuresis could be a result of polyuria with diluted urine production that exceeds bladder capacity. This theory is contradicted by the fact that many children with enuresis have similar urine osmolality as children who do not. For this theory, desmopressin acts as a substitute for endogenous arginine vasopressin. The central question of why these children are not aroused by the sensation of a full bladder is unknown but may be related to the lack of urinary continence skills.

Enuresis is present in 10 to 15 percent of five year olds, 7 percent of ten year olds, and 1 percent of adults. There is a spontaneous cure rate of 15 percent per year after the age of six (Forsythe and Redmond, 1974). Desmopressin therapy has been studied in children as young as six years old, but the best response rates seem to occur in children who are over the age of nine (Post et al., 1983). It is postulated that younger children are more likely to have a developmental nocturnal enuresis due to low functional bladder capacity.

The older child and adolescent who have not spontaneously remitted, more likely lack the diurnal variation in arginine vasopressin.

Most of the desmopressin studies have been conducted in patients with severe enuresis that are unresponsive to other therapies. The criteria for a positive response differs for each study but usually includes the reduction in the number of wet nights (Klauber, 1989; Moffatt et al., 1993). The short-term two- to six-week studies show that desmopressin is better than placebo, with a decreased mean frequency of wet nights ranging from 10 to 91 percent, but short-term dryness is achieved in only 24.5 percent (Moffatt et al., 1993). A 40 mcg dose appears to be more effective, however, one study showed that doses as low as 5 to 10 mcg per night may also be effective (Key, Bloom, and Sanvordenker, 1992). A positive family history for enuresis may be predictive of a positive response to desmopressin (Hogg and Husmann, 1993). Miller, Goldberg, and Atkin (1989) suggest that patients who do respond with complete dryness need three or more months of therapy and tapering the dose of desmopressin by 10 mcg every two weeks may produce a lower rate of relapse. Efficacy of intranasal desmopressin is reduced in patients with upper nasal congestion, allergic rhinitis, or any condition that reduces nasal absorption. Friman and Warzak (1990) state that the negative effects of DDAVP are twofold. First, urine output is reduced and this decreases the opportunity for the child to practice continence skills. Second, the effects of DDAVP last only as long as the drug is taken. In addition, cost is a factor for most families.

Fjellestad-Paulsen, Wille, and Harris (1987), Stenberg and Lackgren (1993), and Matthiesen et al. (1994) studied the safety and efficacy of oral desmopressin. The study by Fjellestad-Paulsen, Wille, and Harris included 30 children aged six to 15 with primary nocturnal enuresis. They compared the effects of 200 mcg of oral to 20 mcg of intranasal desmopressin and placebo. Both routes of administration were equally effective and more effective than placebo. Stenberg and Lackgren studied 24 adolescents, aged 11 to 21, with primary nocturnal enuresis over two 12-week periods. This open study also showed that oral desmopressin was comparable in efficacy to the intranasal route. A comparison of the efficacy of the 200 to 400 mcg oral dose was not given. Matthiesen et al. conducted an open study in 33 children (seven to 18 years old) with monosymptomatic nocturnal enuresis and found oral desmopressin to be comparable to the intranasal route. Two of the patients had an increased response to the intranasal route in comparison to the oral tablets. The authors suggest that some patients who do not respond to one route of administration may respond to the other.

DEVELOPMENTAL PHARMACOKINETICS

Absorption: Absorption from the nasal mucosa is 10 to 20 percent (may be reduced with nasal congestion).
Onset of action: From the intranasal route: one hour.
Time to peak effect/serum concentration: Peak serum concentrations are achieved in one hour, but vary with the rate of intranasal absorption. Plasma levels of DDAVP do not differ between responders and nonresponders (Norgaard et al., 1990).
Duration of action: Variable: eight to 20 hours. The variation may be due to the rate of absorption from the nasal mucosa.
Half-life: The plasma beta half-life has been reported as 3.3 to 4.0 hours in children with diabetes insipidus (Fjellestad-Paulsen et al., 1987). The manufacturer lists a half-life of 75.5 minutes.

DOSAGE RANGES

Primary Nocturnal Enuresis

The manufacturer suggest an initial intranasal dose for children, older than six years of age, 10 mcg or 0.1 ml per naris, for a total dose of 20 mcg intranasally at bedtime. This dose is continued for three days. If there is no response, the dose is increased to 40 mcg. If there is a response at 20 mcg, the dose can be reduced to 10 mcg to check for response to this lower dose. There may be a dose response pattern with higher doses (40 mcg) resulting in more effectiveness (Klauber, 1989), although doses as low as 5 to 10 mcg per night have been effective in one study (Key, Bloom, and Sanvordenker, 1992). The oral doses of desmopressin are ten times the intranasal route; 20 mcg intranasally is equivalent to 200 mcg of oral (Fjellestad-Paulsen, Wille, and Harris, 1987; Matthiesen et al., 1994).

ADVERSE EFFECTS REPORTED IN CHILDREN AND ADOLESCENTS

COMMON

Nasal congestion, transient headache, epistaxis, and mild abdominal pain. (Epistaxis may be associated with the nasal pipette method of administration.)

LESS COMMON

Conjunctivitis, ocular edema, lacrimation, dizziness, asthenia, chills, rhinitis, sore throat, cough, upper respiratory infection, flushing, nausea, vulval pain, and a slight elevation in blood pressure.

ALLERGIC REACTION: Allergic skin reactions may be due to the preservative, chlorobutanol, in DDAVP spray (Itabashi, Katayama, and Yamaji, 1982) and are unlikely due to desmopressin itself. There are very few reports of itching or rash associated with the use of DDAVP (Rhone-Poulenc Rorer, personal communication).

TOXICITY: Signs and symptoms of hyponatremia or water intoxication include continuing headache, decreased urination, rapid weight gain, confusion, drowsiness, seizures, and coma. Desmopressin-induced water intoxication and hyponatremia is frequently associated with excessive fluid intake.

ADVERSE REACTIONS/CASE REPORTS

Low Sodium, Water Intoxication, Subsequent Seizures

Hourihane and Salisbury (1993) reported an eight-year-old healthy girl with secondary nocturnal enuresis who received desmopressin during a camping trip. Twelve hours after the second dose of 20 mcg of desmopressin the child had a generalized tonic-clonic seizure. Upon admission to the hospital the child was confused and uncooperative, with a serum sodium concentration of 119 mEq/L. Later testing showed normal urinary concentrating ability. The child recovered with no further findings. The authors advise cautious prescribing of this drug for nocturnal enuresis.

Bamford and Cruickshank (1989) reported on a six-and-a-half-year old boy with primary nocturnal enuresis who received 20 mcg of desmopressin at bedtime for eight days. Symptoms at the time of admission to the hospital were headache, followed by vomiting, drowsiness, and an episode of seizure-like activity. Subsequently the child was irrational, agitated, and not following verbal commands. The child's serum sodium was 122 mEq/L. The patient was hospitalized overnight and awoke with a slight headache and a serum sodium of 137 mEq/L. The parents reported that they supervised the administration of the drug and gave the boy one puff in each nostril before bed, however if they thought the medication had not gone in properly they repeated the dose once. The parents also observed that the child tended to drink excessively during the daytime. The authors advise that fluid be restricted one hour before desmopressin administration and during the night. They also suggest that excessive drinking during the day be a contraindication to desmopressin therapy (Bamford and Cruickshank, 1989).

Beach, Beach, and Smith (1992) reported on a ten-year-old boy with enuresis who was treated with 20 mcg of desmopressin for two evenings. The next day the child developed repeated bouts of hiccups which he self-treated by drinking water. The patient's mother administered 10 mcg of desmopressin that evening because the patient had been dry the previous evenings. The patient vomited once during the night and in the morning but ate a large breakfast. He later developed generalized tonic-clonic seizures lasting several minutes. The patient's serum sodium was 118 mEq/L. The patient was treated with intravenous saline and was fully recovered in 24 hours. The authors recommend that fluid intake be restricted to 30 ml/kg during the two to four hours before and 12 hours after desmopressin administration. In addition, they recommend against using desmopressin on sleep overs or camp outs, if the adult is unfamiliar with the drug or the child's normal fluid intake.

Simmonds, Mahony, and Littlewood (1988) reported on a 13-

year-old female with cystic fibrosis and recurrent nasal polyps who was treated with 10 to 20 mcg of desmopressin for primary nocturnal enuresis. The patient was concurrently taking intravenous azlocillin and tobramycin. After four doses of desmopressin, the patient developed headache, nausea, and vomiting with a sharp weight gain of 1.8 kg. Serum sodium on the third day of therapy was 125 mEq/L but had decreased to 114 mEq/L on the fourth day. On the fourth day she had a convulsion and subsequently remained comatose. Fluid restriction for 40 hours was followed by intravenous fluids with her normal daily sodium requirement. The patient remained unconscious for 48 hours but gradually regained consciousness over the following two weeks. The authors suggest that desmopressin be used in patients with cystic fibrosis or nasal polyps with great caution.

Hamed, Mitchell, and Clow (1993) reported a ten-year-old boy with primary nocturnal enuresis who was given intranasal desmopressin, 20 mcg at bedtime for two months and then 40 mcg at bedtime for five months. Imipramine 25 mg at bedtime was then added. Two weeks prior to admission he had had a minor head injury. On the day of admission he was unconscious and hypothermic, and subsequently had a tonic-clonic seizure. His serum sodium was 113 mEq/L. The authors indicate the hyponatremia could be a result of the desmopressin, the imipramine, or both. They recommend that the two drugs not be prescribed together and that patients be monitored more frequently while on desmopressin.

Yaouyanc et al. (1992) reported on a 28-month-old child who was treated for high fluid intake, and nocturnal and diurnal enuresis. The child was initially prescribed 20 mcg of desmopressin two times daily. Several days later the dose was decreased to 20 mcg due to vomiting. The child developed anorexia, increased salt intake, and headaches. Six weeks after starting desmopressin the child was hospitalized for a tonic-clonic seizure. Serum sodium was 118 mEq/L. The mother of the child gave the child a drink when he cried and fluid consumption had progressively increased. The child fully recovered. The authors stated that desmopressin was not indicated in this case due to the young age of the child. In addition, fluid intake needs to be monitored by the parents.

DRUG INTERACTIONS

DRUG	DRUGS	EFFECT
Desmopressin	Carbamazepine, chlorpropamide, clofibrate, urea, fludrocortisone	Concurrent use may potentiate the antidiuretic effects.
Desmopressin	Demeclocycline, lithium, norepinephrine, large doses of epinephrine, heparin, alcohol	Concurrent use may decrease the antidiuretic effect of desmopressin.

MONITORING GUIDELINES

Baseline Assessment:

- Rule out other causes of enuresis: Neurologic and/or spinal abnormalities, diabetes insipidus or diabetes mellitus, chronic renal failure, bacteriuria. Check urine for specific gravity, glucose, protein, blood, and infection (Friman and Warzak, 1990).
- Rule out drugs known to cause or exacerbate enuresis: e.g., lithium, antipsychotics.

Time Patterns for Response:

- After dosage adjustments, patients respond to desmopressin therapy quickly and the response is usually not increased with increased duration of therapy. Response is usually rapidly lost after discontinuation of desmopressin.

Follow-Up Assessment:

- Laboratory workup: Check serum electrolytes (especially serum sodium) if therapy is to continue beyond seven days. Check urine osmolality/urine volume and adjust dose; recommended to monitor at (unspecified) appropriate intervals (USP).

Drug Discontinuation: A specific method for discontinuation has not been investigated, however, Miller, Goldberg, and Atkin (1989) suggest that tapering the dose of desmopressin by 10 mcg every two weeks may produce a lower rate of relapse.

INSTRUCTIONS FOR PARENTS/CARE GIVERS/ CHILDREN/ADOLESCENTS

- Administer one-half of the dose per nostril.
- Administer only the prescribed dose. Children may want to take extra doses to "stay dry for sure."
- Store this medication and all medications away from the patient and other children and adolescents.
- For two hours prior to bedtime, drink only enough fluid to satisfy thirst, to avoid water intoxication. Avoid caffeine-containing products.
- Have the child empty their bladder right before bedtime.
- Keep the product tightly capped and refrigerated; do not freeze. The unopened product will maintain stability up to three weeks at room temperature. When traveling keep the product away from extremes in temperature and pack in ice if possible.
- The 5 ml bottle of the DDAVP® nasal spray contains 50 doses of 10 mcg each. Any solution in the bottle after the 50 doses should be discarded. It contains less than 10 mcg per dose. Do not transfer the remaining fluid into another spray bottle.
- Follow the manufacturer instructions to ensure that the drug is deposited properly in the nasal cavity and does not pass down the throat.
- If the child has a cold or nasal congestion, the effectiveness of the medication may be decreased.

PRODUCTS AVAILABLE

DDAVP® Nasal Spray is available in a 5 ml bottle with spray pump that delivers 50 doses of 10 mcg per 0.1 ml metered dose (0.01 percent). DDAVP® contains desmopressin acetate, chlorobutanol as a preservative, and sodium chloride 0.9 percent, and hydrochloric acid for pH adjustment to 3.5. DDAVP® is also marketed in a parenteral product for intravenous injection and as a nasal solution (0.01 percent) that is administered with a calibrated nasal tube.

COST

GENERIC NAME	TRADENAME	AWP*	AWP* per dose
Desmopressin	DDAVP® Nasal Pump	$107.70/5ml	$2.15 per 10 mcg dose

AWP* is the average wholesale price to the pharmacist that is listed in the *1994 Redbook* (Cardinale, 1994).

NALTREXONE

Naltrexone hydrochloride

Trexan® is marketed by DuPont Pharmaceuticals.

DSM-IV INDICATIONS

Autism, self-injurious behavior (???)

Mental retardation, self-injurious behavior (???)

FDA: Safety and efficacy have not been established in children under 18 years of age (*PDR,* 1994).

USP: Appropriate studies have not been performed in patients up to 18 years of age (*USPDI,* 1994).

CONTRAINDICATIONS: Hypersensitivity to naltrexone, concurrent administration of opioid drugs, dependency on opiate drugs, opioid withdrawal, hepatic failure or disease, acute hepatitis.

PHARMACOLOGY: Naltrexone is a relatively pure opioid antagonist that binds to the opioid receptors in the central nervous system. Naltrexone reversibly blocks the effects of opioids. Naltrexone appears to block the effects of the opioids by competitive binding at the opioid receptor. In adults, naltrexone may be more effective in blocking the euphoria than blocking respiratory depression or miosis. The effects of naltrexone are surmountable with very high doses of opioid antagonist. Attempts to overcome the blockade of naltrexone with high doses of opioid agonists is very dangerous and may lead to respiratory depression and death. Although naltrexone is considered to be an opioid antagonist, naltrexone has been associated with several symptoms that are suggestive of opiate agonist effects as well.

Naltrexone appears to have a significant effect on the secretion of the gonadotropins (luteinizing hormone, follicle-stimulating hormone), adrenocorticotropin, cortisol, and catecholamines. Acute dosing of naltrexone is associated with elevations of these hormones that is not found on chronic dosing. Naltrexone appears to have little or no effect on prolactin, growth hormone, thyroid-stimulating hormone, insulin, glucagon, vasopressin, or gut hormones. Naltrexone is also associated with decreased food intake (Atkinson, 1984). The significance of these findings in children or adolescents is unknown.

The effects of naltrexone on self-injurious behavior (SIB) may be related to blockade of the mu opioid receptor. SIB may be a result of beta-endorphin dysfunction which is a mu receptor ligand. Naltrexone may inhibit SIB by reversibly blocking the mu receptor. It is suggested that lower doses of naltrexone may have an effect on the mu opioid receptor while higher doses effect other opioid receptors subtypes, specifically the kappa opioid receptor. The effect of higher doses of naltrexone on the kappa opioid receptor may result in a modification of the mu receptor and result in a loss of effect (King, Au, and Poland, 1993). This implies that naltrexone may have a therapeutic window effect with low doses resulting in a reduction in SIB and high doses resulting in a loss of effect or an exacerbation in SIB (Knabe, Schulz, and Richard, 1990).

STUDIES OF NALTREXONE EFFICACY

Self-Injurious Behavior

Manifestations of self-injurious behavior (SIB) include head banging, self-biting, self-hitting, gouging, and slapping. A biological cause of SIB has not been determined, but may be related to endogenous opioids. In open trials, naltrexone therapy has been associated with a reduction in SIB. There are two hypothesis of how SIB is associated with endogenous opioids. The first hypothesis is that SIB reflects an insensitivity to pain due to excessive basal activity of endogenous opioids. The second hypothesis is that SIB stimulates the production and release of endogenous opioids. Naltrexone, by blocking the activity of the endogenous opioids at their receptors, may reduce SIB.

The clinical effects of naltrexone in the treatment of self-injurious behavior are controversial. Open trials indicate that naltrexone is effective in reducing SIB (Bernstein et al., 1987; Campbell et al.,

1988; Campbell et al., 1989; Leboyer, Bouvard, and Dugas, 1988; Herman et al., 1987; Panksepp and Lensing, 1991) in autistic and mentally retarded children. In addition, double-blind, placebo-controlled case studies involving five patients report positive findings with naltrexone in the treatment of SIB (Leboyer et al., 1992; Walters et al., 1990). Patients appear to have a dose-dependent but individualized response. Lower doses of naltrexone (0.5 to 1.5 mg/kg) were more effective than higher doses (2.0 mg/kg).

Campbell et al. (1993) reported on the behavioral effects of naltrexone in a double-blind, placebo-controlled study of 41 inpatients aged 2.9 to 7.8 years. The level of intellectual functioning ranged from severely retarded to dull-normal. After a two-week placebo baseline period, the children were randomly assigned to placebo or naltrexone for a period of three weeks, followed by a one-week placebo period. Naltrexone was initiated at 0.5 mg/kg/day and increased after one week to 1.0 mg/kg/day. Campbell et al. (1993) reported that naltrexone reduced hyperactivity, but had no significant effect on the core symptoms of autism. Naltrexone had no effect on discriminant learning, and self-injurious behavior (SIB) was not improved. The authors acknowledge that higher doses may have had a more significant effect, but suggest that naltrexone is not a first line agent in the treatment of autism or for those with SIB. Further studies are needed to determine the role of naltrexone in the treatment of SIB.

DEVELOPMENTAL PHARMACOKINETICS

Absorption: In adults, naltrexone is quickly absorbed, with peak blood levels at one hour. Naltrexone undergoes extensive first-pass hepatic metabolism.

Metabolism: Naltrexone is extensively metabolized to several metabolites. The major metabolite is 6-beta-naltrexol. This metabolite is believed to be an opioid antagonist and may contribute to the opioid receptor blockade.

Elimination: Naltrexone and metabolites are excreted primarily by the kidney.

Onset of action: In open studies of children with SIB, the effects of naltrexone were noted within the first hour after administration.

Time to peak effect: The time to peak effect has not been studied, but most investigators assessed the patients for response one to three hours after administration.

Duration of action: In adults, blockade of opioid receptors varies from 24 to 72 hours depending on the dose administered.

Half-life: In healthy adults, the half-life of naltrexone is biphasic. During the first 24 hours the half-life of naltrexone is 3.9 hours. This is followed by a very slow decline in plasma concentrations with a terminal half-life of 96 hours. This long terminal half-life suggests that naltrexone may be sequestered in body tissues and slowly released into the systemic circulation. The half-life of 6-beta-naltrexol is 12.9 hours during the first 24 hours, followed by a terminal half-life of 18 hours. In adults, the pharmacological effects are from 24 to 72 hours and are independent of dose (Crabtree, 1984). Plasma half-lives have not been evaluated in children.

Plasma levels: Plasma levels of naltrexone do not appear to be associated with behavioral response (Campbell et al., 1989).

Self-injurious behavior: In open studies and in one double-blind study, naltrexone is dosed between 0.5 to 1.5 mg/kg/day in children and adolescents. Open studies suggest that naltrexone has a dose-dependent response in the treatment of self-injurious behavior. It is suggested that higher doses (> 1.5 mg/kg/day) are associated with a loss of positive response. Doses of naltrexone should be individualized.

ADVERSE EFFECTS REPORTED IN CHILDREN AND ADOLESCENTS

Preliminary investigations of the side effects of a single dose of naltrexone (0.5, 1.0, 1.5, and 2.0 mg/kg per dose) in "healthy," autistic children indicate that there are no significant changes in cardiovascular function, body temperature, body weight, or serum concentrations of liver enzymes (Herman et al., 1993). In the report by Campbell et al. (1993) the adverse effects in children aged three to eight years old were excessive sedation, decreased appetite, and vomiting. Liver function tests and electrocardiograms were unchanged during three weeks of naltrexone 1.0 mg/kg/day. Naltrexone, when administered in high doses in adults patients, is associated with elevated hepatic transaminase enzymes (Crabtree, 1984). Hepatotoxicity is observed when adult patients receive doses fivefold larger than recommended (300 mg per day). Although the serum transaminases were elevated, the adult patients were clinically asymptomatic, and the transaminases returned to normal in three to six weeks following discontinuation of naltrexone. There are numerous reports of other adverse effects in the adult populations. Additional, long-term investigations are required to accurately determine the adverse effects of naltrexone in children and adolescents.

COMMON

Preliminary information suggests that short-term administration of naltrexone is associated with excessive sedation, decreased appetite, and vomiting (Campbell et al., 1993).

LESS COMMON

Due to the lack of extended treatment studies, there is a lack of information in this area. Practitioners are encouraged to monitor for the adverse effects that have been reported for adults, until further information is available.

ALLERGIC REACTION: Unknown.

TOXICITY: Unknown, possible loss of previous positive response.

DRUG INTERACTIONS

DRUG	DRUGS	EFFECT
Naltrexone	Opoid containing medications, including cough and cold products, antidiarrheal products and opoid analgesics	Naltrexone will block effects of these medications and the patient may not benefit from the opoid containing medications. The blockade effect of naltrexone is surmountable with very high doses

of opoid agonists. Attempts to overcome the blockade of naltrexone with high doses of opioid agonists (e.g., morphine) are very dangerous, and may lead to respiratory depression and mortality. It is necessary to discontinue naltrexone therapy several days prior to elective surgery if administration of opioid agonists is indicated.

MONITORING GUIDELINES

Baseline Assessment:

- History and physical, including weight and height of the patient.
- Liver function tests (serum transaminases, alkaline phosphatase). Other laboratory tests according to patient status.

Time Pattern for Response: The effects of naltrexone have been reported to occur within one hour in open studies. The response to naltrexone appears to be variable and dose-dependent.

Follow-Up Assessment:

- Liver function tests should be monitored monthly for the first six months then periodically thereafter. If significant elevations in liver enzymes occur, naltrexone should be discontinued.
- Monitor for decreased growth as a result of decreased food intake.
- Monitor for additional adverse effects that are reported for adult patients and may occur in children or adolescents, including (but not limited to): skin rash, blurred vision or eye pain, confusion, discomfort while urinating and/or frequent urination, earache, edema, fever, severe abdominal pain, hallucinations, hypertension, mental depression or mood changes, unexplained nosebleeds, phlebitis, tinnitus, shortness of breath, or swollen glands.

Drug Discontinuation: Specific guidelines for discontinuation have not been suggested; however, abrupt withdrawal has been associated with an immediate return in self-injurious behavior in open trials of naltrexone.

SPECIAL INSTRUCTIONS FOR PARENTS/CARE GIVERS/ CHILDREN/ADOLESCENTS

- Notify all physicians, dentists, and pharmacists of the use of naltrexone.
- Naltrexone does not cause physical or psychological dependence.
- If a skin rash develops, stop the naltrexone and check with your physician.
- Store this medication and all medications away from the patient and other children and adolescents.

PRODUCTS AVAILABLE

Naltrexone is available as Trexan® from DuPont Pharmaceuticals. Trexan® is marketed in white, round, scored tablets that contain 50 mg of naltrexone.

COST

GENERIC NAME	TRADENAME	AWP*	AWP* per dose
Naltrexone	Trexan® 50 mg	$439.00 for 100 tablets	$4.39 per tablet

* AWP is the average wholesale price to the pharmacist that is listed in the *1994 Redbook* (Cardinale, 1994).

REFERENCES

Beta-Blockers

Arnold, LE, Aman, MG. Beta blockers in mental retardation and developmental disorders. *J Child Adolesc Psychopharmacology,* 1991;1:361-373.
Cardinale, VA (ed). *1994 Drug Topics Redbook,* Medical Economics Company, Inc., 1994; 235, 256, 274, 345.

Famularo, R, Kinscherff, R, Fenton, T. Propranolol treatment for childhood post-traumatic stress disorder, acute type. *Am J Dis Child,* 1988;142:1244-1247.

Garland, EJ, Smith, DH. Panic disorder on a child psychiatric service. *J Am Acad Child Adolesc Psychiatry,* 1990;29:785-788.

Gillette, DW, Tannery, LP. Beta blocker inhibits tricyclic metabolism. *J Amer Acad Child Adolesc Psychiatry,* 1994;33:223-224.

Grizenko, N, Vida, S. Propranolol treatment of episodic dyscontrol and aggressive behavior in children. *Can J Psych,* 1988;33:776-778.

Kastner, T, Burlingham, K, Friedman, DL. Metoprolol for aggressive behavior in persons with mental retardation. *Am Fam Physician,* 1990;42:1585-1588.

Kuperman, S, Stewart, MA. Use of propranolol to decrease aggressive outbursts in younger children. *Psychosomatics,* 1987;28:315-319.

Kymissis, P, Martin, E. Antistuttering medication. *J Amer Acad Child Adolesc Psychiatry,* 1990;29:840.

Matthews-Ferrai, K, Karroum, N. Metoprolol for aggression. *J Amer Acad Child Adolesc Psychiatry,* 1992;31:994.

Physician's Desk Reference. Oradell, NJ: Medial Economic Data, 1994.

Sylvester, C. Psychopharmacology of disorders in children. *Psych Clinic North Amer,* 1993;16:779-791.

Van Winter, JT, Stickler, GB. Panic attack syndrome. *J Pediatr,* 1984;105:661-665.

United States Pharmacopeia, Drug Information, 1994 Volumes I and II. Sections on beta-blockers.

Williams, DT, Mehl, R, Yudofsky, S, Adams, D, Roseman, B. The effect of propranolol on uncontrolled rage outbursts in children and adolescents with organic brain dysfunction. *J Amer Acad Child Psychiatry,* 1982;21:129-135.

Wyerth-Ayerst, Inderal® Product Information.

Buspirone

Alessi, N, Bos, T. Buspirone augmentation of fluoxetine in a depressed child with obsessive-compulsive disorder. *Am J Psych,* 1991;148:1605-1606.

Cardinale, VA (ed). *1994 Drug Topics Redbook,* Medical Economics Company, Inc., 1994;123-124.

Kranzler, HR. Use of buspirone in an adolescent with overanxious disorder. *J Amer Acad Child Adolesc Psychiatry,* 1988;27:789-790.

Kutcher, SP, Reiter, S, Gardner, DM, Klein, RG. The pharmacotherapy of anxiety disorders in children and adolescents. *Psych Clinics of North America,* 1992;15:41-67.

Physician's Desk Reference. Oradell, N.J.: Medical Economic Data, 1994.

Quiason, N, Ward, D, Kitchen, T. Buspirone for aggression. *J Amer Acad Child Adolesc Psychiatry,* 1991;30:1026.

Realmuto, GM, August, GJ, Garfinkel, BD. Clinical effect of buspirone in autistic children. *J Clin Psychopharm,* 1989;9:122-125.

Simeon, JG. Use of anxiolytics in children. *Encephale,* 1993;19:71-74.

Soni, P, Weintraub, AL. Buspirone-associated mental status changes. *J Amer Acad Child Adolesc Psychiatry,* 1992;31:1098-1099.

United States Pharmacopeia, Drug Information, 1994, Volumes I and II. Sections on buspirone.

Carbamazepine

Baldessarini, RJ, Teicher, MH, Cassidy, JW, Stein, MH. Anticonvulsant cotreatment may increase toxic metabolites of antidepressants and other psychotropic drugs. *J Clin Psychopharmacol,* 1988;8:381-382.

Bertilsson, L, Hojer, B, Tybring, G, Osterloh, J, Rane, A. Autoinduction of carbamazepine metabolism in children examined by a stable isotope technique. *Clin Pharmacol Ther,* 1980;27:83-88.

Birkhimer, LJ, Curtis, JL, Jann, MW. Use of carbamazepine in psychiatric disorders. *Clin Pharm,* 1985;4:425-434.

Brown, CS, Wells, BG, Cold, JA, Froemming, JH, Self, TH, Jabbour, JT. Possible influence of carbamazepine on plasma imipramine concentrations in children with attention deficit hyperactivity disorder. *J Clin Psychopharmacol,* 1990; 10:359-362.

Campbell, M, Gonzalez, NM, Silva, RR. The pharmacologic treatment of conduct disorders and rage outbursts. *Psych Clinic North Amer,* 1992;15:69-85.

Cardinale, VA (ed). *1994 Drug Topics Redbook,* Medical Economics Company, Inc., 1994;127,185,375.

De la Fuente, JM. Carbamazepine-induced low plasma levels of tricyclic antidepressants. *J Clin Psychopharm,* 1992;12:67-68.

Evans, RW, Clay, TH, Gualtieri, CT. Carbamazepine in pediatric psychiatry. *J Amer Acad Child Adolesc Psychiatry,* 1987;26:2-8.

Friedman, DL, Kastner, T, Plummer, AT, Ruitz, MQ, Henning, D. Adverse behavioral effects in individuals with mental retardation and mood disorders treated with carbamazepine. *Amer J Mental Retard,* 1992;96:541-546.

Kafantaris, V, Campbell, M, Padron-Gayol, MV, Small, AM, Locascio, JJ, Rosenberg, CR. Carbamazepine in hospitalized aggressive conduct disorder children: An open pilot study. *Psychopharm Bull,* 1992;28:193-197.

Koivikko, MJ, Valikangas, SL. Hyponatremia during carbamazepine therapy in children. *Neuropediatrics,* 1983;14:93-96.

Kurlan, R, Kersun, J, Behr, J, Leibovia, A, Tariot, P, Lichter, D, Shoulson, I. Carbamazepine-induced tics. *Clin Neuropharm,* 1989;12:298-302.

Pellock, JM. Carbamazepine side effects in children and adults. *Epilepsia,* 1987;28:S64-S70.

Physician's Desk Reference. Oradell, NJ: Medical Economic Data, 1994.

Pleak, RR, Birmaher, B, Gavrilescu, A, Abichandani ,C, Williams, DT. Mania and neuropsychiatric excitation following carbamazepine. *J Amer Acad Child Adolesc Psych,* 1988;27:500-503.

Pynnonen, S. Pharmacokinetics of carbamazepine in man: A review. *Therap Drug Monitor,* 1979;1:409-431.

Reiss, AL, O'Donnell, DJ. Carbamazepine-induced mania in two children: Case report. *J Clin Psych,* 1984;45:272-274.

Sobotka, IL, Alexander, B, Cook, BL. A review of carbamazepine's hematologic reactions and monitoring recommendations. *DICP Ann Pharmacother,* 1990; 24:1214-1219.

Trimble, MR. Anticonvulsants in children and adolescents. *J Child Adolesc Psychopharmacol,* 1990;1:107-124.

United States Pharmacopeia, Drug Information, 1994, Volumes I and II. Sections on carbamazepine.

Clonidine

Allen, DB. Effects of nightly clonidine administration on growth velocity in short children without growth hormone deficiency: A double blind, placebo-controlled study. *J Pediatr,* 1993;122:32-36.

Boehringer Ingelheim, Catapres® Product Information, Drug Information Division, personal communication.

Borison, RL, Ang, L, Hamilton, WJ, Diamond, BI, David, JM. Treatment approaches in Gilles de la Tourette's syndrome. *Brain Res Bull,* 1983;11:205-208.

Cardinale, VA (ed). *1994 Drug Topics Redbook,* Medical Economics Company, Inc., 1994;145-146.

Cohen, DJ, Detlor, J, Young, JG, Shaywitz, BA. Clonidine ameliorates Gilles de la Tourette syndrome. *Arch Gen Psychiatry,* 1980;37:1350-1357.

Comings, DE, Comings, BG, Tacket, T, Li, S. The clonidine patch and behavior problems (letter). *J Am Acad Child Adolesc Psychiatry,* 1990;29:667-668.

Dawson, PM, Vander Zanden, JA, Werkman, SL, Washington, RL, Tyma, TA. Cardiac dysrhythmia with the use of clonidine in explosive disorder. *DICP,* 1989;23:465-466.

Fankhauser, MP, Karumanchi, VC, German, ML, Yates, A, Karumanchi, SD. A double-blind placebo-controlled study of the efficacy of transdermal clonidine in autism. *J Clin Psych,* 1992;53:77-82.

Ghaziuddin, M, Tsai, L, Ghaziuddin, N. Clonidine for autism (letter). *J Child Adolesc Psychopharmacology,* 1992;2:239-240.

Goetz, CG, Tanner, CM, Wilson, RS, Carroll, S, Como, PG, Shannon, KM. Clonidine and Gilles de la Tourette's syndrome: Double blind study using objective rating methods. *Ann Neurol,* 1987;21:307-310.

Harris, JM. Clonidine patch toxicity. *DICP Ann Pharmacother,* 1990;24: 1191-1194.

Harris, JM. Correction: Clonidine patch toxicity. *DICP Ann Pharmacother,* 1991; 25:682.

Huk, SG. Transient exacerbation of tics in treatment of Tourette's syndrome with clonidine. *J Am Acad Child Adolesc Psychiatry,* 1989;28:583-586.

Hunt, RD. Treatment effects of oral and transdermal clonidine in relation to methylphenidate: An open pilot study in ADD-H. *Psychopharmacol Bull,* 1987; 23:111-114.

Hunt, RD, Minderaa, RB, Cohen, DJ. Clonidine benefits children with attention deficit disorder and hyperactivity: A report of a double-blind placebo-cross-over therapeutic trial. *J Am Acad Child Adolesc Psychiatry,* 1985;24:617-629.

Hunt, RD, Capper, L, O'Connell, P. Clonidine in child and adolescent psychiatry. *J Child and Adolesc Psychopharmacology,* 1990;1:87-102.

Jaselskis, CA, Cook, EH, Fletcher, KE, Leventhal, BL. Clonidine treatment of hyperactive and impulsive children with autistic disorder. *J Clin Psychopharmacol,* 1992; 12:322-327.

Kemph, JP, DeVane, CL, Levin, GM, Jarecke, R, Miller, RL. Treatment of aggressive children with clonidine: Results of an open pilot study. *J Am Acad Child Adolesc Psychiatry,* 1993;32:577-581.

Kerbeshian, J, Burd, L. Novel side effects of clonidine in the treatment of Tourette disorder (letter). *J Clin Psychopharmacol,* 1987;7:207-208.

Leckman, JF, Ort, S, Caruso, KA, Anderson, GM, Riddle, MA, Cohen, DJ. Rebound phenomena in Tourette's syndrome after abrupt withdrawal of clonidine. Behavioral, cardiovascular, and neurochemical effects. *Arch Gen Psych,* 1986;43:1168-1176.

Leckman, JF, Detlor, J, Harcherik, DF, Ort, S, Shaywitz, BA, Cohen, DJ. Short- and long-term treatment of Tourette's syndrome with clonidine: A clinical perspective. *Neurology,* 1985;35:343-351.

Leckman, JF, Hardin, MT, Riddle, MA, Stevenson, J, Ort, SI, Cohen, DJ. Clonidine treatment of Gilles de la Tourette's syndrome. *Arch Gen Psych,* 1991; 48:324-328.

Leckman, JF, Detlor, J, Harcherik, DF, Young, JG, Anderson, GM, Shaywitz, BA, Cohen, DJ. Acute and chronic clonidine treatment in Tourette's syndrome: A preliminary report on clinical response and effect on plasma and urinary catecholamine metabolites, growth hormone and blood pressure. *J Amer Acad Child Psych,* 1983;22:433-440.

Levin, GM, Burton-Teston, K, Murphy, T. Development of precocious puberty in two children treated with clonidine for aggressive behavior. *J Child Adolesc Psychopharmacology,* 1993;2:127-131.

Mimouni-Bloch, A, Mimouni, M. Clonidine-induced hyperglycemia in a young diabetic girl. *Ann Pharmacother,* 1993;27:980.

Physician's Desk Reference. Oradell, NJ: Medical Economic Data, 1994.

Pescovitz, OH, Tan, E. Lack of benefit of clonidine treatment for short stature in a double-blind placebo-controlled trial. *Lancet,* 1988;2:874-877.

Rubenstein, S, Silver, LB, Licamele, WL. Clonidine for stimulant-related sleep problems. *J Am Acad Child Adolesc Psychiatry,* 1994;33:281.

Shapiro, AK, Shapiro, E, Eisenkraft, GJ. Treatment of Gilles de la Tourette's syndrome with clonidine and neuroleptics. *Arch Gen Psych,* 1983;40:1235-1240.

Shear, NH, Raddle, IC. Percutaneous drug absorption. In: Raddle IC, MacLeod SM, eds. *Pediatric Pharmacology and Therapeutics.* St Louis: Mosby, 1993: 377-383.

Singer, HS, Gammon, K, Quaskey, S. Haloperidol, fluphenazine and clonidine in

Tourette syndrome: Controversies in treatment. *Pediat Neurosci*, 1985-86; 12:71-74.

Steingard, R, Biederman, J, Spencer, T, Wilens, T, Gonzalez, A. Comparison of clonidine response in the treatment of attention-deficit hyperactivity disorder with and without comorbid tic disorders. *J Am Acad Child Adolesc Psychiatry*, 1993;32:350-353.

Toy, C, Middleton, RK. Clonidine for growth acceleration. *DICP Ann Pharmacother*, 1991;25:1339-1340.

United States Pharmacopeia, Drug Information, 1994, Volumes I and II. Sections on clonidine.

Desmopressin

Bamford, MF, Cruickshank, G. Dangers of intranasal desmopressin for nocturnal enuresis. *J R Coll Gen Pract*, 1989;39:345-346.

Beach, PS, Beach, RE, Smith, LR. Hyponatremic seizures in a child treated with desmopressin to control enuresis. *Clin Pediatr*, 1992;31:566-569.

Cardinale, VA (ed). *1994 Drug Topics Redbook*, Medical Economics Company, Inc., 1994;156.

Fjellestad-Paulsen, A, Wille, S, Harris, AS. Comparison of intranasal and oral desmopressin for nocturnal enuresis. *Arch Dis Childhood*, 1987;62:674-677.

Fjellestad-Paulsen, A, Tubiana-Rufi, N, Harris, A, Czernichow, P. Central diabetes insipidus in children: Antidiuretic effect and pharmacokinetics of intranasal and peroral 1-deamino-8-D-arginine vasopressin. *Acta Endocrinologica*, 1987;115:307-312.

Forsythe, WI, Redmond, A. Enuresis and spontaneous cure rate. *Arch Dis Childhood*, 1974;49:259-263.

Friman, PC, Warzak, WJ. Nocturnal enuresis: A prevalent, persistent, yet curable parasomnia. *Pediatrician*, 1990;17:38-45.

Hamed, M, Mitchell, H, Clow, DJ. Hyponatremic convulsion associated with desmopressin and imipramine treatment. *BMJ*, 1993;306:1169.

Hjalmas, K, Bengtsson, B. Efficacy, safety and dosing of desmopressin for nocturnal enuresis in Europe. *Clin Peds*, 1993;32 (Suppl):19-24.

Hogg, RJ, Husmann, D. The role of family history in predicting response to desmopressin in nocturnal enuresis. *J Urol*, 1993;150:444-445.

Hourihane, J, Salisbury, AJ. Use caution in prescribing desmopressin for nocturnal enuresis. *BMJ*, 1993;306:1545.

Itabashi, A, Katayama, S, Yamaji, T. Hypersensitivity to chlorobutanol in DDAVP solution. *Lancet*, 1982;8263:108.

Key, DW, Bloom, DA, Sanvordenker, J. Low-dose DDAVP in nocturnal enuresis. *Clin Pediatr*, 1992;31:299-301.

Klauber, GT. Clinical efficacy and safety of desmopressin in the treatment of nocturnal enuresis. *J Pediatrics*, 1989;114:719-722.

Knudsen, UB, Rittig, S, Norgaard, JP, Lundemose, JB, Pedersen, EB, Djurhuus, JC. Long-term treatment of nocturnal enuresis with desmopressin. *Urol Res*, 1991;19:237-240.

Matthiesen, TB, Rittig, S, Djurhuus, JC, Norgaard, JP. A dose titration and an open 6-week efficacy and safety study of desmopressin tablets in the management of nocturnal enuresis. *J Urol,* 1994;151:460-463.

Miller, K, Goldberg, S, Atkin, B. Nocturnal enuresis: Experience with long-term use of intranasally administered desmopressin. *J Pediatr,* 1989;114:723-726.

Moffatt, ME, Harlos, S, Kirshen, AJ, Burd, L. Desmopressin acetate and nocturnal enuresis: How much do we know? *Pediatrics,* 1993;92:420-425.

Norgaard, JP, Rittig, S, Djurhuus, JC. Nocturnal enuresis: An approach to treatment based on pathogenesis. *J Pediatr,* 1989;114:705-710.

Norgaard, JP, Jonler, M, Riis-Jorgensen, JC, Christensen, S, Rittig, S, Djurhuus, JC. Pharmacokinetics of DDAVP in treatment of nocturnal enuresis. *J Urol,* 1990;143:218A.

Post, EM, Richman, RA, Blackett, PR, Duncan, P, Miller, K. Desmopressin response in enuretic children: Effect of age and frequency of enuresis. *Am J Dis Child,* 1983;137:962-963.

Physician's Desk Reference. Oradell, NJ: Medical Economic Data, 1994.

Rew, DA, Rundle, JS. Assessment of the safety of regular DDAVP therapy in primary nocturnal enuresis. *Brit J Urol,* 1989;63:352-353.

Rhone-Poulenc Rorer, DDAVP® Product Information, Drug Information Division, personal communication.

Simmonds, EJ, Mahony, MJ, Littlewood, JM. Convulsion and coma after intranasal desmopressin in cystic fibrosis. *BMJ,* 1988;297:1614.

Stenberg, A, Lackgren, G. Treatment with oral desmopressin in adolescents with primary nocturnal enuresis. *Clin Peds,* 1993;32 (Suppl):25-27.

United States Pharmacopeia, Drug Information, 1994, Volumes I and II. Sections on desmopressin.

Yaouyanc, G, Jonville, AP, Yaouyanc-Lapalle, H, Barbier, P, Dutertre, JP, Autret, E. Seizure with hyponatremia in a child prescribed desmopressin for nocturnal enuresis. *J Toxicol Clin Tox,* 1992;30:637-641.

Naltrexone

Atkinson, RL. Endocrine and metabolic effects of opiate antagonists. *J Clin Psych,* 1984;45:20-24.

Bernstein, GA, Hughes, JR, Mitchell, JE, Thompson, T. Effects of narcotic antagonists on self-injurious behavior: A single case study. *J Am Acad Child Adolesc Psychiatry,* 1987;26:886-889.

Campbell, M, Adams, P, Small, AM, Tesch, LM, Curren, EL. Naltrexone in infantile autism. *Psychopharm Bull,* 1988;24:135-139.

Campbell, M, Anderson, LT, Small, AM, Adams, P, Gonzalez, NM, Ernst, M. Naltrexone in autistic children: Behavioral symptoms and attentional learning. *J Am Acad Child Adolesc Psychiatry,* 1993;32:1283-1291.

Campbell, M, Overall, JE, Small, AM, Sokol, MS, Spencer, EK, Adams, P, Foltz, RL, Monti, KM, Perry, R, Nobler, M, Roberts, E. Naltrexone in autistic children: An acute open dose range tolerance trial. *J Am Acad Child Adolesc Psychiatry,* 1989;28:200-206.

Cardinale, VA (ed). *1994 Drug Topics Redbook,* Medical Economics Company, Inc., 1994;392.

Crabtree, BL. Review of naltrexone, a long-acting opiate antagonist. *Clin Pharm,* 1984;3:273-280.

Herman, BH, Asleson, GS, Powell, A, Borghese, BA, Ruckman, R, Fitzgerald, C. Cardiovascular and other physical effects of acute administration of naltrexone in autistic children. *J Child Adoles Psychopharm,* 1993;3:157-168.

Herman, BH, Hammock, MK, Arthur-Smith, A, Egan, J, Chatoor, I, Werner, A, Zelnick, N. Naltrexone decreases self-injurious behavior. *Ann Neurol,* 1987; 22:550-552.

King, BH, Au, D, Poland, RE. Low-dose naltrexone inhibits pemoline-induced self-biting behavior in prepubertal rats. *J Child Adol Psychopharmacology,* 1993;3:71-79.

Knabe, R, Schulz, P, Richard, J. Initial aggravation of self-injurious behavior in autistic patients receiving naltrexone treatment. *J Autism Dev Disorders,* 1990; 20:591-592.

Leboyer, M, Bouvard, MP, Dugas, M. Effects of naltrexone on infantile autism. *Lancet,* 1988;1:715.

Leboyer, M, Bouvard, MP, Launay, JM, Tabuteau, F, Waller, D, Dugas, M, Kerdelhue, B, Lensing, P, Panksepp, J. Brief report: A double-blind study of naltrexone in infantile autism. *J Autism Dev Disorders,* 1992;22:309-319.

Panksepp, J, Lensing, P. Brief report: A synopsis of an open trial of naltrexone treatment of autism with four children. *J Autism Dev Disorders,* 1991; 21:243-249.

United States Pharmacopeia, Drug Information, 1994, Volumes I and II. Sections on naltrexone.

Walters, AS, Barrett, RP, Feinstein, C, Mercurio, A, Hole, WT. A case report of naltrexone treatment of self-injury and social withdrawal in autism. *J Autism Dev Disorders,* 1990;20:169-176.

Index

Abbott Laboratories
  Cylert (Pemoline, Magnesium), 1
  Janimine (imipramine), 41,69
Abdominal pain
  buspirone-related, 208
  clonidine-related, 234-235
  desmopressin-related, 246
  lithium-related, 131,160,173
  naltrexone-related, 257
Abnormal Involuntary Movement
    Scale (AIMS), 125
Acetaminophen, drug interactions
  beta-blockers, 201
  carbamazepine, 221
Acidifiers, interaction with central
    nervous system stimulants, 26
Acne
  clomipramine-related, 51
  as lithium contraindication, 158
  lithium-related, 166,173
  tricyclic antidepressants-related,
    56
Adenylate cyclase, lithium-related
    inhibition, 158
Adrenergic receptors, monoamine
    oxidase inhibitor
    (MAO-I)-related down-
    regulation, 81
Andrenocorticoptropin,
    naltrexone-related increase,
    252-253
Adverse effects. *See also* specific
    adverse effects, e.g., Nausea
  antipsychotics, 123-124,125-126,
    127-128,129,130-131,
    133-140
  benzodiazepines, 181,182,183,
    184-186

Adverse effects *(continued)*
  beta-blockers, 194,195,199-200
  bupropion, 73,76-78
  buspirone, 208,209-210
  carbamazepine, 214,217-220
  central nervous system stimulants,
    20-27
  chlorpromazine, 131,134
  clomipramine, 50,51-52
  clonidine, 227,234-238
  clozapine, 130,134,138,139
  DDAVP, 244
  desmopressin, 244,246-248
  fluoxetine, 91,92,93-94,95-99,102
  haloperidol, 125-126,127-128,
    129,131,134,160
  imipramine, 49,207
  lithium, 131,158-159,160,165-169,
    173
  loxapine, 129
  mesoridazine, 134
  molindone, 134
  monoamine oxidase inhibitors
    (MAO-I), 83,84-85
  naltrexone, 252,253,255-256
  nortriptyline, 46
  pemoline, magnesium, 20-21,23
  pimozide, 127,139
  thioridazine, 139-140
  tranylcypromine, 83,85
  trazodone, 105-106,107-108,110,
    207
Advil (ibuprofen), interaction
    with lithium, 173
Aggression
  antipsychotics-related, 127,138

Bupropion *(continued)*
  drug interactions, 26,78,85
  DSM-IV indications, 72
  efficacy studies, 72-74
  monitoring guidelines, 79
  pharmacology, 72
  special instructions to parents/care givers/children/adolescents, 79
  toxicity, 77
  trade name and generic products available, 72,80
Burroughs Wellcome, Wellbutrin (bupropion), 72,80
Buspar (buspirone), 212
Buspirone, 206-212
  adverse effects, 208,209-210
  allergic reactions, 210
  contraindications, 206
  cost, 212
  developmental pharmacokinetics, 208-209
  dosage ranges, 209
  drug interactions, 210-211
  DSM-IV indications, 206
  efficacy studies, 206,207-208
  monitoring guidelines, 211
  pharmacology, 206
  special instructions to parents/care givers/children/adolescents, 212
  toxicity, 210
  trade name and generic products available, 206,212

Caffeine, drug interactions
  central nervous system stimulants, 26
  lithium, 170
Calcium channel blocking agents, interaction with lithium, 170
Calcium iodide, interaction with lithium, 170

Calcium salts, interaction with beta-blockers, 200
Carbamazepine, 213-225
  adverse effects, 214,217-220
  allergic reactions, 218
  contraindications, 213
  cost, 225
  developmental pharmacokinetics, 214-216
  discontinuation, 223
  dosage ranges, 215,216-217
  drug interactions, 215,220-222, 225
    antipsychotics, 141
    benzodiazepines, 187
    bupropion, 78
    desmopressin, 249
    fluoxetine, 100
    lithium, 170
    monoamine oxidase inhibitors (MAO-I), 85
    tricyclic antidepressants (TCA-D), 61-62
  DSM-IV indications, 213
  efficacy studies, 213,214
  monitoring guidelines, 222-223
  pharmacology, 213-214
  special instructions to parents/care givers/children/adolescents, 224-225
  toxicity, 218
  trade name and generic products available, 213,225
Carbamazepine epoxide (CBZ-E), 215,216
Cardiac disease. *See also* Arrhythmias, cardiac; Cardiovascular symptoms
  beta-blockers therapy, 198
  drug contraindications in, 202
Cardiovascular symptoms
  antipsychotics-related, 133
  beta-blockers-related, 194,195, 196,197,198,199-200

Cardiovascular symptoms
(continued)
central nervous system stimulants-
related, 23,24,28
clomipramine-related, 50,51-52
clonidine-related, 236-237
desipramine-related, 47,48,57-58
lithium-related, 168-169
tricyclic antidepressants (TCA-D)-
related, 55-56,64-65
Catatonia, antipsychotics-related,
136
Catecholamines, naltrexone-related
secretion increase, 252-253
Central nervous system depressants,
drug interactions
benzodiazepines, 186
buspirone, 211
clonidine, 238
fluoxetine, 101
trazodone, 108,110
tricyclic antidepressants (TCA-D),
63
Central nervous system stimulants,
1-39
adverse effects, 20-24
allergic reactions, 24
contraindications, 1
cost, 31
developmental pharmacokinetics,
16-18
dosage ranges, 18-20
drug holidays, 14
drug interactions, 25-27
fluoxetine, 101
monoamine oxidase inhibitors
(MAO-I), 86
over-the-counter products, 30
DSM-IV indications, 1
efficacy studies, 1,3-16
attention-deficit/hyperactivity
disorder, 3-14
comorbidity, 9,10-14
drug combinations, 15-16

Central nervous system stimulants
(continued)
medication placebo trial, 14-15
monitoring guidelines, 27-29
multimodal therapy, 15
pharmacology, 2-3
special instructions to parents/care
giver/children/adolescents,
29-30
tolerance, 9,28
toxicity, 24-25
trade name and generic products
available, 30-31
Central nervous system symptoms.
See also Anxiety/anxiety
disorders; Delusions;
Dysphoria; Depression;
Fatigue; Hallucinations;
Headaches; Insomnia;
Irritability; Mania; Seizures
beta-blockers-related, 194
central nervous system
stimulants-related, 22
tricyclic antidepressants
(TCA-D)-related, 56
Chest pain, buspirone-related, 209
Chlordiazepoxide
as anxiety disorder therapy, 181
contraindication for preschool
children, 180
cost, 191
developmental pharmacokinetics,
183
dosage ranges, 184
trade name and generic products
available, 179,189-190
Chlorobutanol, as DDAVP
preservative, 250-251
allergic reactions to, 246
Chlorpromazine
adverse effects, 131,134
cost, 148-149
interaction with lithium, 169
as low-potency antipsychotic, 123
pharmacology, 123-124

DDAVP *(continued)*
  developmental pharmacokinetics,
    245
DDAVP nasal spray, 250-251
Delirium, antipsychotics-related,
    138,140
Delusions, bupropion-related, 76
Demeclocycline, interaction with
    desmopressin, 249
Depression, 9,10
  antipsychotics-related, 127,138
  anxiety disorders-related, 181-182
  beta-blockers-related, 194,196,
    199,203
  central nervous system stimulants-
    related, 22
  clomipramine-related, 51
  clonidine-related, 235
  desipramine-related, 51
  fluoxetine therapy, 90-92
  lithium therapy, 161
  monoamine oxidase inhibitor
    (MAO-I) therapy,
    81,82-83,84
  naltrexone-related, 257
  propranolol-related, 196
  tricyclic antidepressant
    (TCA-D)-resistant
    fluoxetine therapy, 92
    lithium therapy, 161
    monoamine oxidase inhibitor
      (MAO-I) therapy, 82-83
    tricyclic antidepressant (TCA-D)
      therapy, 45,54,59,69
Desipramine
  adverse effects, 46,48,57-58,60
  as attention-deficit/hyperactivity
    disorder therapy, 46,47-48,54
  cost, 70
  as depression therapy, 42,54
  developmental pharmacokinetics,
    52,53
  as enuresis therapy, 44
  as hyperpyrexia cause, 60

Desipramine *(continued)*
  norepinephrine reuptake-inhibiting
    activity, 43
  as obsessive-compulsive disorder
    therapy, 50-51
  as sudden death cause, 57-58
  toxicity, 42
  trade name and generic products
    available, 41,68-69,70
Desmopressin, 242-251
  adverse effects, 244,246-248
  allergic reactions, 246
  contraindications, 242
  cost, 242,251
  developmental pharmacology, 245
  discontinuation, 249-250
  dosage ranges, 245
  drug interactions, 221,249
  DSM-IV indications, 242
  efficacy studies, 243-245
  monitoring guidelines, 249-250
  oral versus intranasal
    administration, 244-245
  pharmacology, 242-243
  special instructions to parents/care
    givers/children/adolescents,
    250
  toxicity, 246
  trade name and generic products
    available, 250-251
Desyrel (trazodone), 104,110,111
Developmental disorders,
    beta-blocker therapy, 198
Dexedrine, 1,30,31
Dexedrine Spansules, 31
Dextroamphetamine
  as attention-deficit/hyperactivity
    disorder therapy, 82
  contraindications, 1
  cost, 31
  developmental pharmacokinetics,
    16
  dosage guidelines, 18-19
  extended-release dosage forms, 31
  as Fragile X Syndrome therapy, 12

Irritability *(continued)*
carbamazepine-related, 217,220
central nervous system stimulants-
related, 22
clonidine-related, 231
fluoxetine-related, 91
imipramine-related, 49
monoamine oxidase inhibitors
(MAO-I)-related, 88
trazodone-related, 105
tricyclic antidepressants (TCA-D)-
related, 49,67
Isoniazid, drug interactions
bupropion, 78
carbamazepine, 221
Intraconazole, interaction with
bupropion, 78

Janimine (imipramine
hydrochloride), 41,69,70
Jaundice, carbamazepine-related,
217,223,224

Ketocaonzole, interaction with
bupropion, 78
Kindling, carbamazepine-related
inhibition, 213-214
Klonopin (clonazepam), 179,190,191

Lacrimation, desmopressin-related,
246
Laryngeal dystonia, antipsychotics-
related, 136
Learning disabilities, attention-
deficit/hyperactivity disorder-
associated, 9-10
Lederle Laboratories, Loxitane
(loxapine), 121,147,150
Lemmon Pharmaceuticals
Epitol (carbamazepine), 213,225
Orap (pimozide), 122,147

Lethargy
beta-blockers-related, 199
carbamazepine-related, 214,217
central nervous system stimulants-
related, 22
Leukocytosis, central nervous system
stimulants-related, 24
Leukopenia, carbamazepine-related,
217
Levodopa, interaction with central
nervous system stimulants, 25
Librium (chlordiazepoxide), 179,
189-190,191
Lithane (lithium carbonate), 157
contraindications, 158,168
Lithium, 157-177
adverse effects, 131,158-159,160,
165-169,173
allergic reactions, 168
contraindications, 158
cost, 175
developmental pharmacokinetics,
161
discontinuation, 159,172
dosage predictions, 162-164
dosage ranges, 161-162
drug interactions, 169-171,
173-174
antipsychotics, 141
bupropion, 78
carbamazepine, 221
central nervous system
stimulants, 25
desmopressin, 249
fluoxetine, 100
DSM-IV indications, 157
efficacy studies, 157,159-161
monitoring guidelines, 171-172
pharmacology, 158-159
special instructions to parents/care
givers/children/adolescents,
172-174
toxicity, 168,173
trade name and generic products
available, 157,174-175

Lithium carbonate
  cost, 175
  dosage ranges, 162
  trade name and generic products
    available, 157,174
Lithium citrate syrup
  cost, 175
  dosage ranges, 162
  trade name and generic products
    available, 157,175
Lithonate (lithium carbonate),
  157,174,175
Lithotab (lithium carbonate),
  157,174,175
Lopressor (metoprolol), 193,204,205
Lorazepam
  cost, 191
  dosage ranges, 184
  trade name and generic products
    available, 179,190
Loxapine
  adverse effects, 129
  cost, 150
  interaction with central nervous
    system stimulants, 25
  as moderate-potency
    antipsychotic, 123
  as schizophrenia therapy, 128-129
  trade name and generic products
    available, 121,147,150
Loxitane (loxapine), 121,133,147,
  150

Mania
  carbamazepine-related, 217,
    218-219
  fluoxetine-related, 92,96-97
  lithium therapy, 163,171
  sertraline-related, 97
  tricyclic antidepressants
    (TCA-D)-related, 59
Manic-depression, monoamine
  oxidase inhibitors
  (MAO-I)-related, 83

Maprotiline, interaction with
  fluoxetine, 100
Marion Merrell Dow, Norpramin
  (desipramine), 41,68-69,70
Mask-like facies, antipsychotics-
  related, 127,128
McNeil Pharmaceuticals, Haldol
  (haloperidol), 121,147,
  149-150
Mead Johnson Pharmaceuticals
  Buspar (buspirone), 206,212
  Desyrel (trazodone), 104,110,111
Medipren (ibuprofen), interaction
  with lithium, 173
Mellaril (thioridazine), 122,148,
  150-151
Memory impairment. *See also*
  Cognitive dysfunction
  antipsychotics-related, 123,138
  benzodiazepines-related, 185,188
Menstrual dysfunction,
  antipsychotics-related,
  124,140
Mental retardation
  attention-deficit/hyperactivity
    disorder-associated, 9-10,
    12-13
  beta-blocker therapy, 193,196-197,
    198
  lithium therapy, 161
  naltrexone therapy, 252,253-254
Meperidine, drug interactions
  central nervous system stimulants,
    25
  monoamine oxidase inhibitors
    (MAO-I), 81,86
Mesoridazine
  adverse effects, 134
  cost, 150
  as low-potency antipsychotic, 123
  pharmacology, 123-124
  special instructions for parents/
    care givers/children/
    adolescents, 145